BACK FOR SECONDS

THE NOT-SO-DIRTY LITTLE SECRET TO WEIGHT LOSS AND FOOD FREEDOM

CAROLINE MATHIAS

Community with Caroline

Tulsa, OK
https://caroline.fit/

Cover and Layout Design by aspiretodesign.com

ISBN: 978-0-578-98537-4

Printed in the United Stated of America

I dedicate this book to my sister Emily, who not-so-patiently watched me wallow in my own self-destruction for years, and then had to relive it via this book. She is solely responsible for transforming it from a "rambling crackhead's diary" into something "readable."

CONTENTS

INTRODUCTION

For years I joked about being addicted to food, but it was never meant to be a joke. I thought about food all day long, and consequently I allowed it to rule my life as well as my emotional state. In my first book, One More Bite, I talked openly about my struggles with obsessive compulsive disorder, anxiety, anger, and addiction. The need for control when I was at my lowest point led me to alcohol. Things turned dark very quickly and right before my husband and sister stepped in, I decided that I wanted a better life for myself, and for my family. They deserved it, and so did I. So I began a fitness transformation, which changed my life and led me to the revelation that I could not only improve my life, but the lives of others. After years of implementing discipline, focusing on slowly altering my daily habits, making realistic changes, and adopting a "never give up" mindset, I created Community with Caroline (CWC). I want to share my past and my path to a better life with everyone, including you. You are about to read about some of my darkest moments along that journey, how I overcame them, and how you can escape yours, too.

1
CONTROL, ANGER, AND URINE

As a child, I obsessed over and worried about things that none of my friends were concerned with. Most nights, after my parents and sister went to bed, I would sneak out of my room, go into the bathroom, and open and "properly" shut all of the bathroom cabinets and drawers. It drove me nuts and I wasn't sure why I felt compelled to do this, but it was a routine that I had to complete for some time. I was meticulously clean- my room had to be spotless at all times. I spent a lot of time rearranging picture frames so that they were "just so." I would dust until I was satisfied that there was not a speck of dust left. If one of my friends used my makeup, I would wipe it down with rubbing alcohol before using it again. You can imagine what would happen when things were really out of my control!

Aside from this endearing little trait, I also struggled with anxiety, situational depression, and anger issues. My mom used to find me sitting in the living room, cursing at the video games I was playing. I would get so incredibly worked up over the smallest things. When something out of my control would happen, my knee-jerk reaction was to jump to the worst case scenario. When I was in my twenties and one of my friends didn't pick up the phone or immediately call me back, I worried that their unavailability was due to something I had done or that they no longer wanted to be my friend. If I made a mistake on my homework, I would angrily rip up the paper and start over from scratch. I had notes everywhere, and I would rewrite them furiously in perfect handwriting over and over. This is something I still find myself doing, and while I have gotten so much better at it over the last few years, sometimes my irrational anger still is the first to show up to the party.

As a child, these oddities evoked very scary feelings. I never talked about them to anyone because I wanted to appear calm, cool, and collected. I would put on a mask and try to be the coolest chick around, but being gangly and socially awkward made it difficult for me to fit in. Maybe all kids feel like this, but no one I knew was talking about it. We all just tried to make our way through it without being discovered for who we really were.

To compound my awkwardness, when I was in elementary school, I would pee my pants fairly regularly. If someone tickled me too much, I would just start peeing. Neat, right? You can imagine how much fun it was to wet yourself at school and have nothing to change into. I learned quickly how to strategically carry my backpack behind my body so nobody could see the pee stain on the back of my jeans. One day during gym class it happened again. I went to the gym teacher to ask if she had some shorts that I could change into. She was so sweet and helped me into some dry clothes. She also told me that if I wanted to bring a change of clothes up to the school that she would keep them locked up for emergency purposes. So the next day, I brought a spare change of clothes to school, only to find that one of the boys (let's call him "Dick") had found them in my locker before I could discreetly get them to my teacher. Dick threw my clothes in the hallway, right as all of the classes let out. Then, he loudly announced to everyone in the vicinity that the underwear that were laying in the hallway were mine. This was a bright shining moment for me. You know when you have those dreams that you are walking through the halls buck naked and everyone is staring at you? Well, this was what that felt like. I wanted to die. I rushed over to grab the undies and throw them back into my locker. Like most things that suck ass, you just have to keep moving forward, and that is what I did because I'd be damned if I gave Dick the satisfaction he was seeking.

The teasing didn't let up for a while, and I just tried to keep a smiling face, even though I wanted to switch schools and start all over where nobody knew me. As I got older I began playing sports like soccer and softball. I was naturally good, and I enjoyed the competitive aspect of it all. Encouraged by this newfound ability and confidence, I felt powerful for the first time in my life. I wanted to be the fucking best, but I hated it when anyone tried to tell me how to do anything, so coaching me was probably as fun as stabbing yourself in the eye with a pencil. I got really good at soccer, but then kids began picking on me for being good. I was called a "showoff," and that always bothered me. I hated that I felt like I was being punished for being good at something, but this is something I felt like I could control as well. I noticed that if I tried a little less at sports, I was able to make more friends, and the girls were nicer to me in class. So that's what I did. I felt defeated and upset that in order to fit in, I had to change myself again.

* * * * *

Sometimes people come into your life at exactly the right time. The two people who made the biggest impact on my adolescent life were my friends, Katie and Melissa, whom I met the summer before I started sixth grade. They were both very popular and, if you couldn't tell by now, I was not. But we were inseparable from day one, and I felt so much more confident going into a new school with them by my side. I knew this would be my chance to start fresh and make a new group of friends. Hopefully this time around my underwear wouldn't end up on display in the hallway.

I naively thought that middle school would be different from elementary school. The girls would be nicer, right? Ha! Some of the girls were mean as shit, and I never had the wit to bite back. If someone poked fun at me, I just took it. I never said a word to them, but there were plenty of words I'd say to myself. I held onto my anger, and let it fester while I searched for an outlet.

I definitely would not have made it through without Melissa and Katie. During 7th grade, Melissa encouraged me to try out for the cheerleading squad. Being as awkward as I was, I envisioned the judges laughing me out of the tryouts. (Forget tumbling, I still couldn't do a back handspring if my life depended on it!) Filled with self-doubt, I reluctantly tried out. To this day I wonder if Melissa paid them off, but I made the cheer squad, and it ended up becoming a defining moment in my life. I suddenly began to feel cool. I was hanging out with my friends, whom all the boys liked, and I got to be their plus one. However this shift did not mean that teen life was smooth sailing.

I was a late bloomer and very athletic, which set me up perfectly to be the butt of the joke from all the boys. I had rock hard abs and my biceps were huge, so I was nicknamed "beast," "Beowulf," and "beast-o-line." My dad used to make me lift weights three times a week because he didn't want me to get injured playing soccer. I think this period of forced weightlifting is what caused me to develop an aversion to the gym later on in life. The boys would howl at me in the halls, and even though I laughed it off, I was mortified on the inside. I wanted to be looked at the way the other girls were looked at. While the name calling really did bother me, I was finally getting some attention from the boys.

I will never forget the day Melissa and Katie urged me to wear something more girly to school instead of my usual highwater jeans, brown belt with black shirt, and Doc Martens. So, at their advice, I wore a little black dress to school. It was tight, short, and I felt like a girl for the first time in my life. I will never forget the looks and comments I received from the boys. I felt a new sense of power and control. This became another pivotal moment in my life. I experienced the power of my own sexuality. Now I could dress a different way and get the approval I had always wanted, and I didn't give a fuck if it was for my body. I will never forget the looks and whistles from my crushes. I finally had their attention, and it seemed so easy? I was in control, and I believe this was the start of my quest to achieve the perfect physique.

Look, I know what you're thinking- c'mon Caroline, what about the incontinence? Well the pee-pants routine never really came to a complete halt. It happened a few times during middle school and let me tell you, peeing your pants is one million times worse in middle school than it is in elementary school.

* * * * *

Despite this persistent problem, I had some of the best times of my life in middle and high school, but also some of the worst. Entering 9th grade at Memorial High School, I was a cheerleader, soccer player, and all around popular kid. Like most teens, when it came to school work, I loathed every single second of it. I hated listening in class. I wanted to talk to my friends, and I couldn't care less about where the red fern grew. I spent my weekends with Katie and Melissa, sitting on the floor of Melissa's room, listening to Jewel or No Doubt, burning incense, and trying on clothes. It was always just the three of us, and those were some of the best times of my life,

As I was living it up as a freshman, I started experimenting with some of the finer things in life: mainly cheap, 3.2% Oklahoma beer. My friends and I started throwing parties on the weekends, drinking beer, and just being high schoolers. This was the beginning of my relationship with alcohol. We started out slow, wining and dining (think Busch Light and Taco Bell), but with each drink, I noticed my OCD and anxiety slipping away with my conscious thoughts. So I drank more. And more.

Whenever I was drinking, I was able to cut loose and not be so worried about what everyone thought of me. It was amazing. Except for the fact that, unbeknownst to me, I just happen to have an extremely addictive personality, and numbness felt a hell of a lot better than constant anxiety and teenage angst. Right before my senior year, I was looking forward to my last year on the cheer squad and soccer team, prom, and graduation. It was supposed to be the best year of my life, and I was fucking pumped. One night changed all of this.

Katie, who always seemed to be a step ahead of the rest of us, had graduated a year early, and was already off at college at Oklahoma State in Stillwater. Melissa was hanging around with a different crowd, and I was feeling pretty alone. I started hanging out with the younger girls on the cheer squad; we mostly spent our time driving around in my red Honda Prelude, drinking, and going to parties. This specific period of my life is what motivates me to make my son,

Kyler, wait until he's 30 to drive. I made some of the dumbest decisions of my life behind the wheel of that car. I was reckless, I was only thinking of myself, and while I thought the alcohol was making everything better, it was actually making it worse.

One night I pulled up to the school for a dance with my regular passenger in the back seat: a case of Busch Light. Already drunk, I walked into the school thinking I was hot shit. I remember seeing some of the teachers whisper to one another, but I was too drunk to notice what they were saying. Then our security guard at the school approached me and asked me if I would take him to my car. I immediately knew I was busted. That walk was fucking horrifying. I knew this would be bad, just not how bad. He saw the beer in my back seat, so now not only was I drunk on school premises, but I also had alcohol on the property. I was 17. I don't remember what happened that night, but I remember the next day at school getting called to the principal's office. Our principal already had it out for me. He was always riding my ass- mostly about the "skimpy" clothes I wore to school. This was my attitude back then, and it's seeping out right now as I am writing these words. It was always someone else's fault. Never Caroline's fault.

He told me that I was being expelled from school for the first semester of my senior year, and informed me that I would be attending Pershing, a "street school." There was another girl who got expelled with me (we'll call her "Cassandra"). It all felt like a bad dream up until our first day of street school. I don't know what I would have done without Cassandra by my side. Having her made it somehow okay. We had to drive all the way past downtown Tulsa to get to our new school, and we soon found out that the kids who were in there with us had done way worse things than we had. On our first day there, a boy and a girl got caught having sex in the bathroom, if that tells you anything. I was suddenly the model "A" student. I was breezing through my work and making great grades. I just wanted to do my time and get the fuck out of there as soon as possible.

Did I learn my lesson? I wish I could tell you I did. But I didn't. I watched my ass more closely once I got back to Memorial, but I was angry. I was angry at the principal, I was angry at my parents, I was angry at everyone but myself. Placing the blame on others came very easily to me, and I held onto this in the years ahead when I would attempt diet after diet. I never looked at myself to realize that it was me all along who held the power to succeed or not. I blamed my friends (why didn't they love food like I did?). I blamed the diets (they were too tough to stick to!). I blamed my genetics (why couldn't they have blessed me with a rock-hard ass so I wouldn't have to put in any work?). I blamed everything around me, except me, and I was the only one who could actually do something about it. This mindset left me feeling miserable and out of control for years, fighting with food, hating my body, wishing I looked like someone else, and not appreciating any part of Caroline for who she really was.

2

POOH BEAR AND "CRAZY CAROLINE"

I remember the first night I met my husband Josh (more commonly known as "Pooh Bear"). It was the summer before our senior year. I was hanging out with a mutual friend and she took me over to his house. He had his own house, by the way, which we all thought was pretty cool. He was independent, tan, and looked like Ryan Phillippe circa Cruel Intentions, which was my favorite movie at the time. I was attracted to him right away, until he opened his mouth. I remember thinking "Fuck, he's arrogant!" I was immediately turned off. He told my friend that he liked me, but it was a hard "no" from me at that point. However, this didn't stop me from using his house as the ultimate hangout spot, getting wasted, and passing out on his couch each night. I was a real catch.

I had gone a good while without getting into any trouble, so of course I had to remedy that. I was on my way to his house one night and I got pulled over for speeding. For the record, I was going six miles over the speed limit, but I was still breaking the law and, of course, I had a cooler of beer in my back seat. The cop made me feel like a fool, but at the time all I remember thinking was how unfair he was being. He took me to the juvenile detention center, cuffed me, and made me sit in the breakroom, feeling wronged, while a bunch of cops sat around me, eating bagels out of a garbage bag. When he told me my parents would have to come get me, it hit me. Couldn't I just be booked and spend the night in a cell? My parents were nowhere near as hard on me as I would have been on myself (or one of my kids), but being arrested was more serious than getting expelled from school. I made sure to keep my nose clean after this. For a few weeks at least.

I began sneaking out of my parent's house late at night to go stay with Pooh Bear. I was becoming more smitten with him the more time I spent at his house. I began doing anything I could to be around him. And that meant telling my parents that I would be at my friend's house, driving all the way to her house to make the phone call that I was in for the night, and then heading to Pooh Bear's house. Being an inconsiderate asshole came naturally to me- I didn't even have to try! One night when I was staying over, we were all jarred awake by the sound of the phone ringing around three in the morning. The machine picked up, and I heard my mom's voice on his answering machine. FUCK. How did she even know I was here? Did my friend rat me out? I heard her say something about my driver's license being found in the neighborhood, so I jumped out of bed to go check my car. I found my driver's side window bashed in, and my wallet gone. Apparently they had tossed my ID out, and as an elderly man was picking up his morning paper, he found the tiny picture of a spray-tanned teen in his driveway, looked up my parent's number, and called them. My parents were never big on discipline, but this seemed to do the trick. My dad told me that I would be grounded for a whole month, and couldn't leave the house to do anything. I felt like my life was over. I couldn't hang out with my friends, and I couldn't go anywhere unless it was school. This fucking sucked, but I will tell you, it worked.

I was holed up in my room for a month while all of my friends continued to go to Josh's house without me. Once I was free, that was the first place I wanted to go to celebrate. We began seeing each other again, but it wasn't "official," even though I had already picked out my wedding dress in my head. This continued until I turned 18 and officially/unofficially moved in with him.

Operating under the non-existent rules of Josh's house, my weekend drinking became weeknight drinking, and my behavior became more and more erratic. I remember one night we were out with our friends and I thought Pooh Bear was acting weird towards me, so I reactively decided to drink more. I threw a huge fit and tried to leave by climbing through the moonroof of my locked car. I ended up setting the alarm off and everyone scattered in fear that the cops would show up and take us all in for underage drinking. That was the last straw for Pooh Bear. He was over my crazy behavior, and we didn't talk for a while after that, but if you think for one second that your girl was going to give in without a fight, you are dead wrong. Once I set my mind to something (for better or worse), I follow through. This trait has been a thorn in my side, but I think it's also one of my best qualities. Now that I (mostly) focus on being productive instead of being an asshole, the scale typically tends to tip in my favor.

He had no idea what was coming. He was even dating someone else. I didn't care though. He could date anyone he wanted, but I was going to take them all down. And that is what I did. I resolutely imposed myself on him. I would go over to his house even when I knew his other girls would be there. I sat my ass right on his couch and refused to leave. I hung out with his other friends and had the time of my life. I was willing to do this until he either kicked my ass out or came to his senses. I am proud to say that he did eventually come to his senses and dumped all the other girls for me. I knew from day one that we were going to end up together, even with his sassy ass attitude. We were finally officially dating, and more importantly, I had gotten my way yet again! There was just one problem-neither of us had officially met "Crazy Caroline" yet.

*****

Like most teens in their first serious relationship, everything felt magical. I loved being around him. He was so fucking sure of himself, so sure of everything it seemed. He made me feel safe. He knew how fucking crazy I was, and he loved me anyway. We were never "best friends" (I hate when couples say that), but we never fought about anything either. To sit here twenty years later and tell you that we have not had hard times in our relationship would be a lie. We have gone through what any normal couple goes through: times where we don't speak, times where we want to kill each other, arguing about how often we should have sex (spoiler alert, he wants it more often than I do). But regardless of all of the hard things about marriage, I know now more than ever that he is the person for me. It just works. Little did I know then, and despite all of the wonder of a new relationship, I was about to enter one of the darkest periods of my life.

After moving out of his high school house, we lived in a condo with a friend for a few years, and then got our very own house. It was great, finally living on our own without a bunch of people coming and going. I had him all to myself! We formed a new friend group with my high school best friend Katie and her husband Daniel, both of whom had just finished college, and spent all of our ample, pre-kids, free time with them. Josh was building a successful landscaping business and told me that I didn't have to work if I didn't want to, which was music to my ears, because I didn't want to. This is when things got really out of control.

I quickly settled into a routine of setting an alarm for 10am, throwing sweatpants on, and driving to Taco Bell. I would get two orders of Nachos Bellgrande, no beef, no beans, extra sour cream, extra cheese, extra tomatoes, and extra jalapenos. I will remember that order until the day I die. I would go home, sit on the couch, read tabloid magazines with perfect women smiling from the covers, turn on The Skulls, and gorge myself. This went on for almost two years. Never in a million years did I expect to divulge this behavior to anyone. It was my dirty little secret, and I loved every second of it.

Up until this time of my life, I had always been skinny. I had never had to think twice about what I was going to eat. Until now. The weight started packing on. It was slow enough that at first, I didn't even notice it. My clothes weren't fitting, yet I still didn't realize what was happening. Josh came home from work one day and asked me if I had eaten Taco Bell again. He was starting to notice. Having someone outside of the reality I'd created where it was just me and Taco Bell call me out, I started to feel shame. I began hiding the bags in the trash can, underneath the other trash, so I could keep my little obsession going. I assured him that I'd cut back, but I didn't.

At this point, I was struggling to fund my habit. I was taking money I found around the house and buying shitty food with it. As hard as it is to admit, I know I can't sugarcoat this behavior. My weight started increasing, and I began to feel even worse about myself- but still not bad enough to stop. It was an addiction. I loved the feeling of eating for the first few minutes, and then I instantly plunged into despair, shame, and guilt each time I finished a meal. Our sex life suffered because I hated myself, plain and simple. I wanted the bad feelings and weight gain to stop, but I was unwilling to give up the one thing causing all of the trouble: binge eating. My food demons had slowly taken control over every aspect of my life.

Looking back on all of this now, I see it so much more clearly. The obsessive compulsive behavior I'd experienced as a child had morphed into obsessing over food. And when the insecurity and shame became too unbearable, the alcohol was there.

3
ALCOHOL

Alcohol was a mask for me. Just like in high school, I was using it to come out of my shell at parties and social gatherings, so that I could be more fun, less boring. I used it to numb feelings that I didn't want to feel, and I went all in, every time. I wanted to take the pressure off and remove my filter. I was fairly well known as a crazy, fun, drunk girl who would do just about anything. I would get so hammered that I didn't give a fuck what came out of my mouth. Charming, I know. But this was my attempt to silence Crazy Caroline and introduce people to the Caroline I knew was inside of me, and who I wanted them to know: Fun Caroline.

Having an obsessive personality had elevated my drinking from a regular high school student, to one who would bring beer to school and drink in the parking lot at 8am. My dad had a "beer" fridge in our garage, and I started taking beer out of it every morning to drink before class started. It made me feel so good on the weekends, why not add it into my weekly rotation? Drinking became a part of who I was, and it lasted all the way up until I began my transformation six years ago. If you were worried that I would gloss over the messy stuff, rest easy. The drinking was the catalyst to my life changing, so it can't be made pretty.

For a while, I was Fun Caroline- to everyone except my sister Emily. Emily always knew the real me, and drunk Caroline was not her. She saw right through me, so she was never fun to have around when I was trying to have a good time. I am completely unable to be reasoned with when I am drunk. She would immediately get annoyed with me and want to leave, knowing that if she didn't get out early, I would continue acting like an asshole with my friends, and she would spend the entire night running damage control, and then sitting with me for hours while I was sick and swearing I'd never eat Taco Bell or drink again. Even if she did manage to leave, I would call her in the middle of the night when no one else wanted to deal with my ass and spend countless hours that I don't remember being reassured by her. We spent a lot of years fighting over my drinking, and I have said some horrible things to my sister that I wish I could take back, but even on the nights when I was the most out of control, I knew that this was not the person I wanted to be. But how could I be anything else? Alcohol made me feel so great, so light. I stopped caring what other people thought of me, and that feeling alone was enough to keep me hooked.

I rarely drink anymore, and the reason is that, no matter how much I would argue the fact, I am not a "fun drunk." Early in our marriage my drinking was very troublesome. It caused way too many late night fights. Alcohol literally removes the good parts of me and ushers in this heinous bitch who is so incredibly self-serving that she scares even me. Emily and Pooh Bear are fun drunks. They get nicer, more talkative, and more enjoyable to be around. I am the exact opposite. I feel great the first few hours, and then a light switch gets turned off, and I am instantly ready to go home. This made me a very difficult person to be around or to take out to fun places. My mood would change at the drop of a hat if alcohol was involved.

Another thing that went out the window with the alcohol was the tenuous hold I had on my diet. On the nights we would go out partying, I had to stop somewhere, usually Taco Bell, on the way home. It was a nonnegotiable, and everyone around us knew it. It was like clockwork: everything would start off fine, and then between drinks 4-6, Crazy Caroline would come out, fly off the handle (usually towards Pooh Bear), and then demand to be taken to Taco Bell and then home, even if I had just eaten. People would always do it because it was easier than dealing with my meltdowns if they didn't. I would eat until I was sick to my stomach, and then pass out.

Like with food, I never have any interest in drinking just a few beers or cocktails. If I was drinking, I was drinking to get drunk. What was the point otherwise? My attitude of all or nothing applied to every aspect of my life. If I was eating, I was binging. If I was thinking, I was overthinking. If I was drinking, I wasn't socially drinking, I was drinking with an agenda. (It's not-so-ironic to me, now that I have built a successful business, that I have a very hard time not overworking.) When you have an all or nothing outlook on life, nothing ever really satisfies you. Have you ever felt satisfied after binging on food? Do you ever wake up with a miserable hangover wishing you had drank more? When you overthink, does it ever solve anything? No. You never reach any level of happiness. I didn't know what I was searching for, but I knew that I wanted to feel important. I wanted people to look up to me. And nobody did. I was the butt of the joke for so long in my group of friends. I spent so long creating Crazy Caroline that she was the only version of me that people (outside of my sister and husband) knew. I had become her, and I couldn't escape her. Nobody took me seriously, and I knew I had to rewrite my story. So I did. It all started with one step: quitting drinking (for a while at least).

*****

After the birth of my daughter, I suffered with postpartum depression (PPD), and naturally I figured my friend alcohol would definitely help with that! With my hormones being out of whack, feeling more alone than I have ever felt in my life, struggling to make it through each day with two young children, dousing the situation with alcohol was, unsurprisingly, a recipe for disaster.

I switched from beer to liquor and wine and began popping wine corks around 1-2pm each day. The first few glasses were heaven, and when the feeling began to fade, as it always does, I would make dinner, gorge myself, go to bed, and wake up to do it all over again. Brynn was a very tough baby; she cried nonstop. It didn't matter what we were doing, she was fucking pissed about it. Being at home with a rambunctious 4-year-old and a screaming baby proved to be a challenge for me, even outside of the PPD. That time in my life was really fucking hard, and I never talked about it to anyone because I felt that I would be judged for airing my frustrations. I feel like anyone who struggles with OCD will inevitably struggle when they have children because you lose control of the things that make you feel safe. Keeping a clean house, having laundry done, those things made me feel sane and now that's out the window! Compounded by the postpartum depression, I did all I knew how to do to feel good and get through each day: drink.

The drinking was obviously not helping, but I couldn't see that at the time. As time went on, a few glasses turned into a bottle (or more) a night, and I began a vicious cycle of self-loathing. Unable to watch me spiral any further, my husband and my sister stepped in and told me that something needed to happen before it got any worse. These two will forever be my people. They know the real me, and at this moment they knew exactly what I needed. A push. My husband had been encouraging me to hire a trainer, and I knew that the moment had finally presented itself. It was now or never. Knowing myself, I knew that if I could just fucking do it, just execute the plan, I could have a new life. And I was right.

After committing to quitting drinking and working with a trainer, I went on the hunt for validation. Validation from everyone who had laughed at me, second guessed me, or underestimated me. Most of us want validation from others. It feels fucking good. But the ultimate validation can only come from yourself. When you are the only one who can approve of you, you win. You no longer need anyone else's approval. You no longer need food to feel a certain way. You no longer need alcohol to make you "less of you and more of someone cooler." You no longer live your life for anyone else but you, and nobody can take that away from you. I finally feel like I am getting closure on my relationship with alcohol. I still drink on occasion, but never anymore to escape my reality. The reality that I have created for myself is too amazing. I don't ever want to escape it.

4

DIET CULTURE

My guess is that 100% of you have tried a fad diet at least once in your life. The very first fad diet I tried was the very popular "no food, run like hell" diet. I simply stopped eating and started doing a shitload of sprinting, even when it was ninety degrees outside. This led to almost passing out, blood sugar spikes and drops, dizziness, and exhaustion. I dropped a little weight doing this, but as you and I both know, this is not a sustainable way to lose weight. It is however a great way to expedite death. Not eating was hard as fuck for me, especially since my every waking thought was of food. This type of deprivation would inevitably lead to full-blown gorge sessions of crap food. When I was a new mother, we started hanging out with other couples with young kids, and I desperately wanted to keep up with my new, thin friends. I wanted to look and feel better about myself, especially when I was around all these stunning women who seemed to have their shit together so much better than I did. Comparison is the thief of joy, and I certainly let it rob me of any joy I could have had during those years. The phrase "Keeping up with the Joneses"? That was me. And it was a losing battle. I was fighting with myself, I was in silent competition with my closest friends, and it was awful.

I've never had an issue with being open about my struggles, which has proved to be good for me in the long run, but back then it was not one of my best qualities. Instead of just working through stuff, I always confided in my friends about it. Financial struggles, marital struggles, arguments--nothing was off limits. It was always Caroline sharing her shit and then feeling less than because they couldn't relate to what I was talking about. I was so used to depending on others to make me feel happy that I never once gave myself the chance to fill that role. This exposed a lot of selfish thoughts and behaviors. I blamed my friends for not having the problems I had, not understanding what it was like for me, and would lash out at them when I would get drunk and my filters were gone.

After failing at eating chicken and rice and running myself into the ground, I hit a point where I was ready to try almost any "quick fix" to look better. I decided I would give HCG a try. HCG (Human Chorionic Gonadotropin) is a hormone injection paired with an incredibly restrictive, no-carb diet. Someone I knew had done it and lost 20lbs in one month, and I didn't know what that acronym meant, but they had me at "lost 20lbs in a month." I started giving myself injections into my stomach and eating just 500 calories per day, every day. Super great for my body, hormone levels, overall well-being, I'm sure. I look back and feel like a moron for doing this. At the time, I just thought, "desperate times call for desperate measures." This is when I first began to realize that the obsession to become "perfect" was not teaching me anything. I was taking these random, drastic measures to achieve the perfect body, to be the perfect person, but I could never just do something without going a thousand miles an hour. If I was on a diet, I wouldn't eat one Dorito, and if I was off my diet, I was eating 8,000 Doritos. I was unaware that a massive shift in my focus would have to take place for me to get out of this hell. A bigger part of the problem is that I was convinced that the more drastic a diet was, the better results I would have, so I was fully complicit in making myself fucking miserable for however long I needed to get the results that I wanted.

I still remember choking down ground buffalo and broccoli with zero seasoning when I was on HCG. It was miserable. After the first successful round, and 24lbs lighter, I was ready to keep the momentum going! I was told I had to refrain from sugar or carbs to keep my new bod, and I remember the words coming out of my mouth before I could even stop them: "Are ya fucking kidding me?" No sugar or carbs, like, ever? This is exactly what is wrong with diet culture, the belief that you must deprive yourself and be miserable to obtain results. I see women on social media brag about how much chicken and rice they eat on a daily basis (humble moment right here, folks; this used to be me), and how many hours they slave away in the gym, and it is just perpetuating a sick idea of what "real' women need to do to achieve their dream body. It's fucking insanity. It wasn't until recently that I discovered that true, lasting results are not achieved by being perfect, but by finding something that works for you that you can actually <gasp> enjoy. But as you probably already know, I had a few more trials to go through before I figured that out.

*****

I am an introvert. I don't get my energy from spending time around large groups of people; I enjoy my quiet time alone more than I enjoy processed nacho cheese. However, I love connecting with people regarding food and their issues with food. The first thing I ask when I meet someone is what their favorite food is. I can talk about food for hours—the trashier the better. I want to know where you find the best fake cheese, the best types of nachos, the best buffalo wings with ice cold bleu cheese dressing. Damn, now I'm hungry.

An obsession with food goes hand-in-hand with an obsession with body image. Almost every single client I've worked with who struggles with body image issues also struggles with food issues as well. And as a result of these struggles, we all look for the easy way out. What can we do to drop weight the fastest? What is the easiest route to rock hard abs? This is how we nose dive into the pit of fad dieting. We are conditioned to think that there must be a level of suffering in order to achieve beauty. If not, it won't work. This is a lie.

Society wants you to believe this so that you will continue to purchase their diet teas, their waist trimmers, their 30-day cleanses; the list goes on for-fucking-ever. These things give you false hope that you can achieve true results in a matter of weeks or months. They say: "Be miserable, trust us, it will work and you will finally love yourself! All for just $19.99!" And I get it. It's tempting. I've been there and done it. All of it.

I spent too much of my life stifled by the judgment of others, worrying about whether or not I would fit into certain groups. I spent years wasting money on things I didn't like. I bought material things so that I could fit in with my friends. I spent so much time acting a certain way to hide "Crazy Caroline." The funny thing is, a lot of people liked Crazy Caroline. And I made her sit in the backseat for years. I put a different version of me in the driver's seat, only to end up continuously disappointed in myself and not pleasing anyone. I spent years being utterly miserable in an attempt to transform my body into something that I thought everyone would want. I went as far as competing in a bikini competition (which I discuss at length in my first book). You know, the ones where you basically deplete your body of all nutrients and water a few days before you stand on a stage to be judged by people you don't even know? My body was the fittest it had ever been, surely this would make me happy! But after taking last place in the open category, and feeling like the hardest work I had ever done was all a waste of time and energy, my first reaction was: "When can I compete again?" My obsessive tendencies were rearing their ugly head once again, and I wanted to win. All rational thoughts were out to lunch. I was consumed by my emotions. I was furious, enraged, indignant.

Thankfully my coach stopped me in my tracks and asked me a question I was not prepared to answer. He asked me why I wanted to win. I told him, "I don't know. I want to win. I feel like I will be happy if I win." He assured me that winning wouldn't make me happy, and then asked me what would make me happy. That was when I knew I was lost. After all of the fad diets, after overcoming PPD and alcohol addiction, after over a year of the hardest training of my entire life, I couldn't answer him. Hearing him tell me that winning wouldn't solve all of my problems devastated me, and left me questioning everything. What would I do now?

The realization that I didn't know what I wanted was more than I could handle. I work so well when I have something to complete. I work until it's done, even if it means working late into the night or at the crack of dawn.

The one and only thing I could answer with certainty was that I was fucking done eating that way.

I wanted a break from eating seven meals of chicken and rice every day. I wanted to go back to enjoying my one true love: nachos. Finally I told him that I no longer wished to diet the way I had been, and that I wanted something to make me feel alive when I woke up every day. Just saying those words were freeing, even though I still had no idea what they meant or why I'd said them. I just knew with certainty that killing myself with competition-level diet and exercise was not it. After years of feeling lost, and finally achieving my perfect body, I had to face the shocking reality that it had not solved all of my problems. I knew it was time to find out what would truly make me happy.

A few years after I began my fitness journey, I began getting dozens of messages daily from women, asking how I had achieved this body I was rocking. I didn't have the strength to tell them that being miserable was the key to having it. I went on about discipline and how just sticking with it was what they needed to do, as if it was this easy. Nevertheless, I began revealing my exact process with the women reaching out to me privately. I wasn't sugarcoating anything. I told them every single thing I did regarding workouts, types of food I was eating, and how difficult it really was, and they respected my honesty. I felt alive sharing my story with them. Speaking about my failures and learning from them falls right off my tongue. It was never forced. It was the first time in my life that something truly appealed to me. So I kept sharing my story, the good, bad, and ugly. During this time, I went on my "post-competition" diet, where I remained focused on maintaining a certain number of macronutrients each day while significantly scaling back my workouts.

Out of every diet I've tried, it's the only one that has worked, kept me consistent, and that I've enjoyed. It's similar to Weight Watchers in that it keeps you within a certain caloric range, but instead of focusing on overall calories, it focuses on the three macronutrients: protein, carbohydrates, and fat.

Protein is so important for fat loss, and most diets don't include enough of it. Protein keeps you feeling satiated longer, so it helps to curb cravings. It speeds up recovery after strenuous exercise, aids in building lean muscle which is necessary for fat loss, and it also helps reduce overall muscle loss.

At Community With Caroline, we believe that life is meant to be lived, and not in a perpetual cycle of diets. We do not guilt or shame our clients for eating any type of food, and we don't allow them to guilt or shame themselves for going over on their macros, or indulging in foods that bring them joy. Our coaches teach our members tips and tricks so that, on days they want to splurge, they can do so without sacrificing progress. As long as they hit their protein all day long and save up their carbs and fats, they can enjoy whatever they want at dinner (within reason). We also focus on mindfulness when it comes to overall portions. These two winning combinations help them stay on track and more importantly stay sane.

PRACTICE

Instead of focusing on what you aren't doing, or how many workouts you didn't get in, start focusing on the things that you did do. Stack those small victories! The key to any form of success are the little things done every single day for an extended period of time. Nobody ever lost 50lbs overnight. Nobody ever started a successful business in a week. It's a marathon. Once that sinks in, you will begin to relax. Find something that works for you and do it over and over and over.

A lot of people enter their fitness journeys with false beliefs that create barriers to success. **Make a list of foods that you have restricted, thinking that if you eat them they will blow your progress:**

1.____________________________________

2.____________________________________

3.____________________________________

4.____________________________________

5.____________________________________

6.____________________________________

7.____________________________________

8.____________________________________

9.____________________________________

10.____________________________________

Another barrier to success is the "too busy" excuse. **Check off some things below that you struggle balancing in your own life.**

___ Kids

___ Marriage

___ Work

___ School

___ Fitness

___ Money

___ Self care

___ Housework

___ Family

___ Friends

Now that some of our false beliefs are laid out, let's talk about our victories. I tell all of my clients to celebrate small victories, and we share them in our Facebook Community.

Weekly Questions to Answer (if you answer one to any of them, that's a victory!):

1. How many workouts did you do? ______________________

2. How many days did you follow your meal plan? _________

3. How many days did you practice self care? _____________

4. How many nice things did you think about yourself? ________

5. How many compliments did you give? ___________________

6. How many times did you journal? _______________________

7. How many times did you meditate, ground, or sit in silence?

____

8. What are some things that made you feel good internally about yourself?

____

5

REPROGRAM, REPEAT

For years, if I was overwhelmed, I did nothing. If I was inspired, I tried to do everything. In between days were not acceptable. This rolled over into the way I viewed my fitness journey. I thought that I had to workout for a minimum of two hours a day for at least five days a week and eat certain things or I wouldn't lose weight. I thought that if I ate carbs after 6pm, they would go straight to my thighs. I stared in the mirror every day and nitpicked my lower tummy area, my cellulite, every inch of my body that wasn't "perfect," and self-sabotaged myself with negative thoughts. I didn't stand a chance. Nothing improved because I was focused on perfection, and perfection isn't real. I thought that nothing was worth doing if I couldn't do it perfectly.

If I could go back in time I would shake myself until that message fell out of my head. Once I started reprogramming my thoughts, the game changed. I started with silencing the negative thoughts about my body the second I recognized myself thinking them. If I headed to the mirror in my bedroom to lean over and see how much my stomach hung over my pants, I turned around and said "we aren't doing that today." It was hard as fuck. It didn't happen overnight, and truthfully, I still work on it. But I can tell you that I rarely stand in the mirror and speak negatively to myself anymore. What is the point? It doesn't fix or change anything. I have also given myself grace regarding my workouts. I no longer feel the need to exhaust my body beyond its capabilities day-in and day-out. Most importantly I acknowledge that it's okay to rest.

Even when I started counting macros, I obsessed over the numbers. Now, I'm not as concerned about hitting my macros perfectly. This is part of the journey that

I wasn't ready for even just a year ago. It has taken me time to learn what to eat on a daily basis. I practiced daily by plugging my numbers in, and once again I remained consistent. The more I did it, the easier it became. Once I got to a point where I realized that as long as I am getting an adequate amount of protein and watching my portion sizes, I knew enough about my macros that I could begin to eat intuitively. For me, eating intuitively was the pot of gold at the end of the fitness rainbow, and tracking macros led me there. And I can tell you honestly- it was worth all of the work. This year has been the first year that I finally feel free. I feel free to be who I truly am. I feel free to eat what I want, when I want, and if I don't track my macros for a few days, I don't beat myself up. This has been a long time coming. It's taken lots of learning, mistakes, and work, but I am in the best position I could have imagined; a position where I can help others do the exact same thing. If you are reading this right now and wanting help, I want you to email me immediately at hello@caroline.fit.

Whenever I get new clients, they are understandably overwhelmed. They've spent years on complicated diets and workouts that ultimately failed. If I could ask you to latch onto one lesson from the beginning, it would be this: don't overcomplicate this. Keep it simple. If you don't like something, change it. If you are mentally abusing yourself, try to catch yourself in the moment and stop it. If something isn't working, stop doing it. Each time you have a setback, reprogram and repeat. If you do these things long enough, they will become your new normal and they won't seem so hard anymore. You are in control of how your life unfolds, starting with your body, your family, your job, your happiness, and the way you view food.

This can be an especially tough lesson for those who feel the need to constantly be everything to everyone. Boy am I guilty of this. I am a type A personality who gets an orgasm each time I mark something off of my to do list. Sometimes this trait serves me, and well, sometimes it really doesn't. I joke that if I never got married or had kids that I would be the crazy lady sitting around de-pilling every pair of socks that I owned and removing specks of dust by the second. Frankly I am getting turned on just thinking about that. I can exhaust myself trying to be

100% at all aspects of my life, knowing that it isn't realistic or attainable, yet I keep trying. One of my clients told me that we cannot be 100% in our marriage, 100% at our jobs, 100% with our children, 100% with our fitness goals, etc. It just doesn't work. Talk about a buzzkill! What's the point of trying then? The need to be perfect still plagues me every single day. I feel most accomplished when I check off every single thing on my to do list, and then some. In a perfect world, on a perfect day, my perfectionism would have me checking off all of the following boxes:

✓ Wake up early

✓ Clean the kitchen (dirty dishes in my sink give me hives)

✓Do a couple loads of laundry

✓ Pick up/declutter the house

✓ Drink some water (warm lemon water first thing in the morning is great for your digestive system!)

✓ COFFEE

✓ Walk outside and do my grounding

✓ Visualize/manifest my day as well as my life. I speak out loud the things I want in my life. Some current examples are:

✓ My second book is a best seller (the one you are reading at this very moment!)

✓ My family is healthy and happy

✓ I lead a Community of 10,000 women

✓ I have five coaches under me with full client lists

✓ I am debt free

✓ Wake my kids up and get them ready for school

✓ Get ready for the day (more often than not this means tossing my hair in a clip and throwing some workout clothes on)

✓ Drop kids off at school (after breaking up a fight in the car about who called whom a "butthole")

✓ Head to my office and crush work goals

✓ Eat (order) lunch

✓ Get to the gym and try not to work while I'm working out

✓ Finish my workout just in time to pick up the kids from school (if my husband hasn't already)

✓ Race home to enjoy time with my family

✓ Get home and try not to think about work stuff

✓ Make/order dinner

✓ Chat with kids and Pooh Bear about their day

✓ Dinner, shower, bedtime

✓ Grown-up time with my husband (I won't act like wife of the year here because this definitely isn't a nightly ritual, but I do my best)

✓ Check on kiddos, lay with Kyler and practice spelling, talk about our fave books, aliens, etc. Then I head to Willie's room. She enjoys talking about farts, frogs, and dinosaurs. I read her a book, smooch her on the forehead and head back downstairs

✓ Once everyone falls asleep, my time begins. This is why I stay up so late. I get to dick around on my phone while watching Austin Powers all by myself with nobody telling me what to do. I used to beat myself up about "not being productive" during this time or "being lazy" because I chose to just check out. I realize how ridiculous this sounds as I type the words, but this is what really goes on in my brain.

That about sums up my idea of a "successful" day, but most of my days don't look like that. Some days my kids need 50% of me, so my husband gets 10%, my business gets 35%, and I get 5%. But I will tell myself the same thing I tell my clients: take each day as it comes. Know that they won't all look the same. You won't hit your macros perfectly every single day. That's okay, keep trying. Just because one meal is a shit show doesn't mean the rest of the day has to be that way. If you don't make it to the gym at all this week, you won't experience a massive setback. I promise. Workouts are 10% of the process, and food is the other 90%. Write that down. Give it your best each day, and recognize that some days the percentages might be a little off.

6

KISS

KISS is a badass rock band, but it also stands for "keep it simple, stupid." My dad used to say this to me as a kid, and I'm sure he is reveling in the fact that I now say it to my clients (respectfully). Why is it so hard for us to keep things simple? If they aren't tough or complicated, why do they not feel like a victory when you achieve them? I hear the same question weekly from dozens of clients: "Why can't I just do this? I overcomplicated it this week, and I failed."

Newsflash! You are not alone. I overcomplicate things to give myself an excuse for not doing what I know I need to do. Some of my favorite excuses for falling off track are, "my week was too stressful," "my job kicked my ass," "I just had too many things going on," and an old standby, "I was pmsing." I felt like if I had a legitimate excuse, I didn't have to put the work in. Problem solved! Only I was cheating myself out of results. When I had the realization that my trainers were not affected in the slightest if I fell off my plan, I suddenly began to care a whole lot more about staying on track, and in order to stay on track, I had to keep it simple. I didn't need a brand new menu or brand new workouts every week. I didn't need brand new resistance bands before I could try the brand new glute workout I found on Instagram. The trick is to find a menu that works for you, and stick with it. I'm not saying you have to eat the same things every week for the rest of your life. I switch up my menu about every 5-6 weeks. I find things that I like and I keep them in my weekly rotation until I get tired of them. I find that it is much easier for me to stay on plan this way.

The same goes for your workouts, and this may crush a lot of souls, but stop switching up your workouts! You don't need "X's Booty Blaster 2000" to build your ass. You need progressive overload, performing the same compound movements over and over each week, focusing on getting stronger and better over time. This is how you will build muscle and burn fat more efficiently, as opposed to extreme cardio and hopping between different and random workouts. Simple isn't exciting, and it sure doesn't sell, but it is the secret. Find what you like, and what works, and stick to it. Changing up your workout all the time overwhelms you and forces you to quit altogether. When it's too much, we shut down. When it is doable and enjoyable, then we can execute.

How I keep it simple:

- Plan my weekly meals every Sunday

- Get groceries that are quick and easy to have on hand and require zero prep

- Pre-log my meals into MyFitnessPal (this makes it SO easy to stay on track each day!)

- Do what you can with the day you have right in front of you. Do not worry about yesterday or tomorrow, they aren't even real. All you have is this moment right now.

- Journal about what you truly want for yourself and your life. Too many times people think they know what they want, but they really don't. Journaling and checking in with yourself is a good way to figure that out.

- Don't overload your plate! If you've got a busy day at work, don't stress about going to the gym! This one is hard for a lot of people, but just giving yourself a break can make you feel lighter almost instantly.

- There is always more time. There is always a new day, a new week. You don't have to be it all today.

- Don't obsess about having to eat a certain amount of meals each day. Do what works with each day that comes. If you eat five meals today, and two tomorrow- great!

Even if you only do two or three of these things each day/week, you're still working towards your goals.

A frequent question I get from my clients is, "How do I quit complaining and just do it? How do I remain patient while waiting for results?" For the record, I complained the whole way through my transformation and was impatient as fuck. The bottom line is that nobody is ever ready for a transformation. Just like we are never fully ready to raise children. It's hard as hell, nobody tells you about the rough days, and persevering sometimes feels impossible. But you gotta keep going (especially when it comes to raising your kids). When I decided that it was time for a real change, I was five months postpartum, drinking every day, eating pure shit, and hating my body. I asked my husband to take some pictures of me so that I could see what I needed to see. I truly didn't recognize myself. Body dysmorphia, a distorted view of your body, is a very real thing. Most women think they look worse no matter what they actually see in the mirror, but I experienced the exact opposite. I thought I looked way better than the pictures showed, and at that moment I knew I was ready. So to answer the question almost all of my clients bring to me, I'll tell you what I told myself in that moment: "Shut the fuck up and just do the work for the first time in your life." Was it easy? No. I complained more than I ever have about being on a diet, having to go to the gym, etc. I begged my husband to explain to me how I was supposed to do this for the rest of my life since it was so miserable. He told me that once I started seeing results, it would make me want to keep going--and dammit, he was right. So I am going to steal his words and use them for my benefit here. Once you do this long enough, and start seeing real changes in your body, you will want to keep going.

This does not mean you won't be miserable on some days, but you can still enjoy what you eat on a daily basis and reach your goals at the same time. Let's be real, nachos are the only thing that consistently kept me going the past six years, not chicken and rice.

I've had many, many setbacks that I will share with you, and the only thing that was really consistent about my journey was my complaining, but the only reason you are reading this book is that I never quit. If you take nothing else from me, take this advice: don't quit. You can fuck up as many times as you want. You can fall off track for a week, two weeks, hell two months, but as long as you never completely quit, you will continue to succeed--at anything.

Results take a long time, and often we are the last to see them. I did not sit by patiently and wait for my results. It's especially hard these days when we can have anything we want with a swipe of a finger. Our instant gratification machines and timelapse videos of success stories make it even more difficult for women to understand that real progress takes time. You didn't gain 40lbs overnight, and you are not gonna lose them in 30, 60, or even 90 days. If being patient is key to making progress, why not make the process as enjoyable as possible? This is where our Community philosophy comes in. This is why we removed all restrictions, guilt, and shame from the equation. To achieve success physically, you need to be consistent and you need to be patient. So in order to make this process easier for you, we want you to enjoy it. If donuts bring you joy, and you are allowed to eat a donut every day on your "plan," you are more likely to stick with that plan consistently for a longer period of time. You may still feel impatient, and even frustrated, while waiting for progress, but we don't beat ourselves up for those feelings. It is all part of the process. When you are feeling impatient, remember that consistency is key and then go indulge in something that will take the edge off. Then get right back on track! Keep doing this and you will never have a problem reaching your goals.

7

DO HARD THINGS

I am eager to follow up that last chapter about giving yourself grace and not focusing on perfection with this chapter: do hard things. I always lead with grace with my clients because that is how I learn best. However, I consider myself a pretty damn good motivator because I have pushed myself beyond my limits time and time again, and I know what my clients are capable of. If you take the "don't give up" advice and decide to take one more note from me, it would be this: just fucking do it. If you don't want to workout, just fucking do it. If you don't want to eat your prepped meal, just fucking do it. If you don't have energy to have sexy time with your husband, just fucking do it. If you don't want to crawl out of bed to go read for an extra ten minutes to your kids, just fucking do it. Noticing a theme yet?

I definitely don't always want to get out of my warm ass bed to go read to my kids, but when I do it is the most rewarding thing ever. I know that they won't be this little forever and I don't want to miss those moments. I don't always have the bandwidth to initiate sexy time with Pooh Bear, but when I do, he always appreciates it and that is rewarding. I definitely don't always want to go to the gym, but I've never gone and felt worse. And I sure as fuck don't always want to stick to my planned meals, but when I do I feel like I could conquer the world. The self confidence that discipline breeds is unlike anything else I have ever experienced. It is so incredibly hard in the moment, but if you can remember each time you are tempted (for me it's about 1,000 times a day) that it only takes five minutes to eat that meal, I promise you will make the right decision. Remember, if it were easy, everyone would do it.

Diet and exercise are not sexy- they are mundane. It's like laundry and dishes; they have to be done. Look at your workouts and meals like that as well. Do I want to empty the dishwasher twice a day? Fuck no, but I have to or we won't have any clean dishes. Do I want to do laundry? Fuck no, but if I don't we won't have clean clothes to wear. Do I want to chug my egg whites every morning? Fuck no, but I want to get a head start on my protein intake for the day. Do I want to go workout or would I rather pick up cheese fries and eat in my car while watching a movie? I'll let you answer that one. But I have made a habit to drive to the gym every day over the past seven years and now it is just what I do. I don't think, I just do. And so should you.

You will never regret working on yourself and your family. With my family is my most favorite place to be. It's where I feel safe. Once you begin working on you, you suddenly realize what you will put up with, and more importantly, what you won't. You will start standing up for yourself, and making decisions based on what you really want. This is crucial. As women it's so easy to lose ourselves as we mature. Whether it happens in school, in marriage, or even as new moms. I spent my entire existence hiding my rage, acting happy when I wasn't, and trying to fit in so hard that I lost who the real Caroline was. I definitely feel like this contributed to my confusion as I hit my twenties. I didn't know who I was, only who I was trying to be. Now that I am 38 years old (it only took me 3.5 minutes to calculate my age), I just want to be me, and I really don't care who accepts me for it or not.

I tossed out most of my old high heels, my designer bags, most of my makeup, and damn near all of my jewelry a few weeks ago when we were packing. Being someone you aren't takes a lot of damn energy, and as you get older, energy is very important! Not giving a fuck about what people think about me has been the best decision of my life. I'm now the person I want to be. The Caroline who will carry the same Freddie Mercury purse for the rest of her life, the Caroline who will never wear heels again (sorry, Pooh Bear), the Caroline who has four items of jewelry, and most importantly, the Caroline who only needs validation from herself. That is the best feeling of all.

*****

I used to drive around town and daydream about owning land, a farm, and lots of animals, of having a certain physique, of being financially stable, but I never really thought I would achieve any of these things. I was in my own way for so long, telling myself so many lies about why I couldn't acquire any of this, that I believed these things would always be just a dream. Now, they are my reality, and I am going to tell you how to create exactly the life that you want. The secret formula is very complicated. All it will take is:

1. Belief that you can do it

2. Work

3. Patience

That's it. It is the boring shit that you have to do, day after day. I have wanted to give up at least 1,000 times over the past six years, but I haven't. I kept moving, even on the days I wanted to curl up into a bag of Doritos (which I did, often). I didn't always believe in myself. Hell, I am not really having a great "believing in myself day" today. But I am forcing myself to sit here and write. I'm not always patient. In the words of Queen, "I want it all, and I want it NOW."

Six years ago I committed to working on myself. I stopped at nothing. I created a new lifestyle. I was working out twice a day, seven days a week, eating very strictly and rarely cheating on my diet. I felt great, I felt in control, and nothing could stop me. I rode this train for a while. When I decided to compete in a bikini show, I started having girls reach out to me for support on their own journeys, asking me questions about which supplements to take, what foods to eat for abs, what workouts to do to "shred." My answers were and always will be blunt and not glamorous: hard fucking work and lots of fucking patience. Nobody wants this formula. They want the quick fix they think you are hiding in your back pocket and keeping from them.

But I wasn't. I was doing the mundane. I was actually shocked at how simple the formula was. Eat less than you burn on a daily basis, and just remain consistent? So why the restrictions then? That was my burning question. I asked this question over and over and none of my coaches would ever give me an answer that made sense. It was like when you're a kid and your mom says "Because I said so!" If calories are calories, why can't I eat donuts? Because sugar. What does sugar do? Makes you fat. Why can't I eat fries? Because fried food makes you fat. I could not accept these answers because they made no sense to me. Ultimately, no food can make you fat. Eating an excess of any food can, but cheeseburgers are fine in moderation. Wine is fine in moderation. Cinnamon rolls are fine in moderation. Chips are fine in moderation. Anything is fine in moderation (except nacho cheese).

But for those just getting started, all you have to do is eat less than you burn on a daily basis. Start here. Follow this one step if you do nothing else. The foundation to this basic formula is protein. Any other crazy rules that a diet tries to impose on you is just a waste of time and energy. At the end of the day, those rules won't derail you if you break them. Over the past six years, I have figured out a formula that works, and I have passed it along to all of the members of Community with Caroline. They eat what they want, when they want, in moderation. That's it. We don't overcomplicate food. We teach our clients how to follow macros. This is the tool to food freedom. Macro-based eating gives you the guidance and freedom to make this way of eating work for you. One of the most important aspects of achieving food freedom is the importance of letting go of the guilt and shame you've attached to eating certain foods. Eating a donut isn't bad. The shame you impose upon yourself for eating that donut is bad. The guilt you feel for eating something you truly enjoy is bad. Food is not bad. Food is not good. Food is food. Once you understand this your life will change and food will no longer have control over you.

Once I started sharing my real life transformation success story with women, this unique relationship began. I started a Facebook group called "Raw, Real, and Spectacular" (a nod to Seinfeld). It was my space to share beauty, workout, and food tips. I would go live in the Facebook group frequently and simply share what was on my mind. During one of those live videos, "Food Demons," I spoke out loud for the first time ever about how I used to binge and hide food. I spoke about the guilt and shame I felt about doing this. More women reached out to me after I did that video than ever before. They told me they had done those same things but never told anyone. I suddenly felt compelled to share more of my "shit." This first Facebook group was a safe place for me to be open and honest about my struggles. It helped me as much as it helped them. I loved it. I became addicted to logging on and being with them, even at six in the morning. It was all I wanted to do. Deep down I began to wonder how I could make this my job.

The problem was that I didn't know how to turn it into a business yet. It was around this time that I ran into a friend I had grown up with. He very bluntly asked me why I was providing all of this knowledge and support online for free. I told him that I didn't really know what I was doing, and that I didn't feel qualified to make money off of it. He began building me up and making me believe that I absolutely could make a business out of this. It took a lot of reassuring conversations, but over time I began to believe that this could be something I could actually do. I started "Community with Caroline" in December of 2017. It began as a 30-day challenge, and I was terrified that nobody would sign up. Since I already had a platform with my Raw, Real, and Spectacular group, I began posting in there about this new group "Community with Caroline," and I had twenty girls sign up that first month for my first challenge. I was so excited! I knew how to write a meal plan, but I still didn't know how to not be restrictive about it. I was still learning that for myself. What changed the game was sharing every aspect of my process with them. I didn't hide anything about it or act like I had it all figured out, because frankly, I still don't.

I will never forget the morning I made a particularly vulnerable video. It was a Monday morning, and I was fresh off a weekend bender. I had fucked the whole weekend up. Ate myself into oblivion. How the hell was I supposed to go live and motivate these women if I still couldn't control myself around food? What came out of my mouth that morning literally changed the course of the Community forever, as well as my life. I spilled the beans. I told them not to worry if they had binged over the weekend, that it was more important not to shame themselves, that it didn't matter what or how much they ate, it mattered that they let it go. It was cathartic even for me to hear these words come out of my mouth. I couldn't stop. I kept pouring out support. Support that I desperately needed to hear as well. The response was insane. I had multiple girls reach out to me, telling me they were crying listening to me tell them not to verbally abuse themselves for "cheating." I removed the word "cheating" from my vocabulary that day. Words like "diet," and "cheat meal" have become toxic to women, specifically. From that moment on, the Community had a vibe, a purpose. I knew I wanted to dedicate the rest of my life to building it, growing it, and reaching as many women as possible to encourage them on their journeys to loving themselves and dropping the guilt, shame, and negative self-talk surrounding their bodies.

I was making some extra money with my challenges while still working full time at my husband's lawn company. I hated my job. Getting yelled at by customers about their grass wasn't really my idea of living the dream. I wanted to feel fulfilled, and this Community made me feel professionally fulfilled for the first time in my life. I wanted this to be my full time gig, so I followed my own advice. I believed this was my calling, I dedicated myself to putting in 100% effort at it every day, and I remained patient. That last part was tough, as I still have massive fucking goals for this Community that I haven't reached yet, but I will. You can bet on it. I started the Community almost three years ago with 20 girls, and today we have over 2,000 members. My short-term goal is 5,000, and my long-term goal is to have a CWC client in every state. But most importantly, I want to empower you, even right now as you are reading my words:

- Never give up. You can do anything you want to.
- Put in the work. Most days, it sucks. Just do it anyway.
- Be patient.
- Repeat.

PRACTICE

Change Your Narrative! Here you will write down statements about yourself/ life that you wish to become a reality. You must write these statements down as if they have already happened or are already this way. Doing this reprograms your brain to believe these as truths, and then it literally works to make them a reality.

Example: If you are a reactive individual, write down "I am not reactive." If you worry, write down "I don't worry about anything." If you want to work for yourself and quit your job, write down "I own my own business."

1.____________________________________

2.____________________________________

3.____________________________________

4.____________________________________

5.____________________________________

6.____________________________________

7.____________________________________

8.____________________________________

9.____________________________________

10.____________________________________

8

THE CHOICES WE MAKE

I promised my community that I would give them the dirt in this book, and I intend to fulfill that promise. This is something that I never planned on sharing with anyone. When I told my sister about it, she said, "If you ever do anything that stupid again, I will kill you with my bare hands." I discussed it with my best friend of 25 years, and she told me that it was something I should never share with anyone, because people will inevitably judge me for it, and she didn't want to see me get hurt. I felt the same way for a few years, but as my story continues to unfold, I think the most authentic thing for me to do at this stage would be to share the shit. Because I share everything. I have built my business on being true and transparent with my clients; they respect that, and they are able to learn from it. So here it goes.

I took steroids.

I sometimes still can't believe that I did it, but I did. I knew what I was doing was wrong, but I was blinded by desperation for something that would catapult me to an even more perfect physique. I knew other women who had done it, and they seemed to be fine, so I convinced myself that I wouldn't be affected. If they had no side effects (or at least none that I was aware of) and I was going to do such a small dose, then surely I would be fine.

You know that moment when you do something and you're immediately aware that you can never return to your old self again? I remember that feeling as I jabbed the needle into my arm that first night. I felt dirty. It felt so wrong. But what happened a few weeks after that first shot seemed to make it all worth it. I saw insane muscle growth in a matter of weeks. My body seemed to function so much better in regards to building muscle and being able to process protein more efficiently. My adrenals and hormones, not so much.

In the beginning I noticed little to no side effects; it seemed too good to be true. Most women, if they had one wish, would wish for the ability to eat everything they want and never gain an ounce of weight. If you don't believe me, turn to your wife or girlfriend and ask her, I bet you that is her answer. That is what was happening to me. I was eating medium pizzas and showing up to the gym the next day with a full six pack of abs. It was like the pepperonis were morphing into little ab muscles. Was this real life? Why had I waited so long to do this? Why is it so taboo? Why don't all girls do this? The more muscles I saw, the more it fueled me in the gym. I remember finally feeling "good enough." I had waited my entire life for this feeling. All of that hard work I had put into fad dieting could have been solved with a little needle in my arm once a week?

I was able to push through the toughest workouts, I was eating tons of food, and my body was immediately turning it to muscle. The first few weeks I spent waiting for the other shoe to drop, to feel "wrong," but it just felt right. However, by week three, I began noticing that I felt super tired every afternoon. So tired that I could barely keep my eyes open on the couch. The tiredness would sometimes carry over into the next day and I would have to take a full day off of work, just to rest. I wasn't drinking enough fluids either, so I was experiencing pain in my lower abdomen, which scared me, but not enough to do anything about it. When I started the cycle, I wanted to be sure that I was doing the lowest dose possible. I wasn't "hardcore," so I wanted the very smallest amount if I was going to do it at all. I heard the false justifications pouring out of me: "You're not even going to do enough to experience any side effects," while my gut was telling me not to do it. But I ignored my gut and listened to other people around me, and now I am paying the price for it.

My voice began to crack. I already have a deeper voice for a woman; it's one of the things about me that my husband has always been attracted to. He said I sounded like a real girl. Well, it's a good thing he didn't want a wife with a high-pitched voice, because mine was cracking and getting deeper by the day. I ignored this charming side effect because--muscles! Even as I type this I am angry with myself all over again.

So I've got the big muscles, I've got the abs, and I can pretty much eat whatever I want and not gain an ounce. I can handle a little exhaustion and crack in my voice if this is the payoff! But as I continued the process, the exhaustion became worse, and soon I began having trouble peeing. My pee was extremely yellow and it was becoming painful each time I had to go. Worst case scenarios began to race through my mind. I probably shouldn't have googled it, but I did. I spent hours mindlessly scrolling worst case scenarios, convinced I was in kidney failure, trying to assure myself I hadn't done enough of it to cause any real damage. But the voice, the exhaustion, and the urination problems weren't enough to make me stop. What, you ask, was the breaking point? One large, black hair sprouting on my chin.

I stopped immediately after plucking that thing from my face. It was too much. My mind was racing: "This isn't fair! I am doing the smallest amount possible and getting every horrible side effect as a result! Why me?!" I can almost hear your sympathy through the page as you're reading this. Boo-fucking-hoo. My sister's voice was in my head, saying "You chose to do this, ya fucking idiot!" And I know. I have moved on from a place of being extremely embarrassed about doing this to my body, to a place of wanting all women to know what really happens when they take extreme measures to achieve a better body. I thought that things would return to normal once I stopped, but they didn't. My voice never came back, I experienced severe adrenal fatigue for almost three years after stopping, and that black hair still comes in, a constant reminder of my choices.

Another crippling side effect of stopping was that going to the gym went from something I loved doing, and considered a privilege to do, to my own worst nightmare. I couldn't workout at any level without feeling like I had the flu for days. All I wanted to do was workout, and I couldn't even do that anymore. It stripped me of everything. Not to mention the mental side effects that take place when your body is readjusting. The one that stings the most, that I have to live with for the rest of my life, is that I can no longer sing. If you know me, you know that music is my life. I used to take long drives, just to sing at the top of my lungs in my car; it was my therapy. I can't do this anymore. The high notes don't come out. I can't scream. It is awful. It is a daily reminder of what I did. I also have a throat clearing reflex that happens at night when I lay down. It is not something that I can't live with, but it is just annoying enough that it disrupts my bedtime every single night.

These are things that I never imagined living with before and now they are a part of my life forever. If I had known that any one of these things would happen, I would never have done it. The hardest part is accepting that these are a result of something that I voluntarily chose to do. So if you are reading this and pondering something drastic, please, please, please learn from my mistakes. The quick and easy route is never worth it. If it is easy, assume that it will come with strings attached. I try not to live my life with regrets, but if there is one thing I could take back, it would be this. The results didn't last, just the side effects, and I can promise you, it wasn't worth it.

9

SETBACKS

While I still experience a lot of guilt for willingly causing myself every setback that came with the steroids, there have also been physical setbacks that I had no control over that threatened my progress, and ultimately, my business. I've experienced three major injuries that have left me with a deep gratitude for a functional body. When I had my ability to workout taken away from me, it became all I could focus on. Being injured taught me so much about myself. Each time I experienced an injury, I had been taking the gym for granted. This attitude led me to put half-ass effort into my workouts, and consequently put my body at risk for injury every single time.

The first injury happened about four months into my transformation. I was on the horizontal leg press machine at the gym when I felt and heard a loud "pop." I immediately flipped out, knowing that what I had just done was not only bad, but that I couldn't go back in time ten seconds, concentrate on what I was doing, and undo it. I immediately stood up, and tried to do a pop squat. Nope, not happening. I limped out of the gym and started bawling my eyes out in my car, while spiraling mentally. "This was it," I thought, "This was the moment that would rip all of my progress away from me. My time was done. It had to end sometime, right? My diet would turn to shit now that I wasn't able to workout. My motivation would dwindle and I would never recover." I had pulled a ligament, and it would take 7-8 weeks to fully heal. After a great pity party, do you know what I did? I didn't quit.

For the first time in my life I didn't give up just because I hit a roadblock. This was huge. I continued going to the gym each day and doing what I could, which was mostly upper body. Guess what? I still made progress. Was it slower than what I had been making? Yes, but here's the kicker: if I had said "Fuck it" at that very moment, I would still be in the same boat I had been in my whole life. Bitching about my body and never making any real changes. But I had been down that road too many times before. This time I kept moving. Once I was fully healed, I felt invincible. I took my workouts super seriously and no longer took them for granted. That first injury taught me that you can absolutely still make progress without giving it 100% every day in the gym. Being able to train is absolutely a privilege and it's important to remember that, especially on off-days.

About a year after my first injury I was sitting at the seated cable row, and I felt something pop in my upper neck and immediately froze. I couldn't breathe. If I tried to breathe the pain radiated throughout my neck. I limped out of the gym and called Pooh Bear. I was freaking out. How the fuck was this happening again? When will you learn to just pay attention when lifting, Caroline?! I was terrified. I went to the chiropractor and luckily it wasn't as bad as I had expected, but I was out for a few weeks again. At this point, my daily habits that I had created over the past 18 months are what kept me on track. So another tip I want to give you is that the longer you implement something into your daily life, the easier it becomes to make that action a habit that is hard to get derailed from. Consistency is boring, but it's what works, not eating Nachos Bellgrande every day and wishing away the fat cells. You can trust me on that- I gave it the old college try for decades.

My third injury changed who I am as a coach, and how I handle myself in all situations to this day. My second neck injury happened when I was taking steroids; it was not an immediate pop like the two previous injuries. It began hurting one evening and felt really sore. I worked out (like an idiot) the following day, pushing through to make sure I had the best body in all the land. I was doing hyperextensions and immediately felt it worsen. I stopped my workout and left the gym. As the day went on, it got worse and worse. I was on such a roll with my physique that this time I was not allowing an injury to take me down. I refused to stop working out. My husband laughed at me as I told him these things. When he suggested I take a week off training, I screamed "Not happening!" at him, but the following days were terrible. I could barely move my neck at all without scorching pain shooting down my back. I couldn't sleep without pain. I suddenly realized that every single movement I made took neck support. One Saturday afternoon, I was sitting in a chair with an icepack on my neck, and I told my husband I was going to the gym to workout. I drove to the gym despite his warnings, crying from the pain. I got on the treadmill and hiked the incline up to 15 and tried desperately to just walk on the treadmill. It was excruciating, but I'm a stubborn asshole, and I wasn't going to take this lying down.

At about minute three on the treadmill I realized that I was fighting a losing battle. I ended up having to take a few months off from doing almost anything weighted in the gym, which meant my roll was over. I had finally hit a groove and now the wind was knocked out of me, once again. I knew deep down that this was necessary, but I didn't know why yet. To this day I am grateful for my neck injury because it taught me that my form is the most important thing in the gym, and I began to research and work on perfecting it so that I could prevent further injury. This would also help me to be a better coach. It suddenly wasn't just about me. I had to coach my girls through their setbacks, and I had to now take the advice I was giving them--to keep going and just do what they could. This, on top of stopping the steroids, was a huge shift, and it was tough to accept at the time.

Some more common setbacks that my clients often cite include kids, family, school, work, life changes, tragedy, sickness, etc. Sometimes these things can toss a wrench into your meal plan/focus/motivation, but you have to get used to working them into your schedule because they will always be there. Embracing setbacks before they happen helps soften the blow when something unexpected comes up, and also helps you to navigate it better because you were prepared mentally. Always remember this: no matter what situation you face, you always have the choice of what goes into your mouth at every single meal. I have lots of clients who are realtors, teachers, nurses, sales reps, etc., and they all say the same thing when they sign up: "I can't eat five meals a day, I just don't have the time. Also, I am out at restaurants multiple times each week and there is almost always alcohol and fried foods involved." My response? Great! You can eat once a day, or eight times a day. It doesn't matter as long as you hit your macros. Also, you can absolutely stay on track, even if you eat at a restaurant every single day. There are always healthy options. Now I get it, I am human too and I know how difficult it is to sit down at a restaurant with a group of people ordering queso, chips, nachos, buffalo wings, etc., and then proceed to order fish and vegetables. So here is one of my most helpful tips for situations like this: eat the damn food.

You heard me. I tell my clients this every single time. If they preload protein and save up all their carbs and fats for dinner, they can partake in any of the foods they want to without falling way off track. This still takes work, but you can absolutely have your nachos and eat them too. So before you get all worked up about having too many work events, upcoming vacations, parties, or Sunday buffets, always remember that the quicker you learn to navigate those situations, the quicker you move to a place of living and loving your life while still making progress. It is possible, but it still takes discipline and planning. After all, who wants to sit at a restaurant and watch people dunk buffalo wings into bleu cheese while you choke down butterless vegetables? Not fucking me.

Another tough setback can be getting out of your routine. Everyone wants to figure out a routine that works, but it needs to be one you can stick to. Most people thrive on a routine, but you better toss this one out the door now. I let this get the best of me for years until I finally just conceded. If my gym routine fell off, it broke me. I would obsess about what went in my mouth or I would binge as a result of not making it to the gym six days in a row. If I messed up one meal on my plan, that meant a full-blown who-gives-a-shit-fest until the following Monday. Instead of just adapting and continuing on like normal the following day, I allowed one tiny setback to screw up and stall my progress for days. This was a choice! You have to expect setbacks. Expect breaks in your routine. There is always tomorrow. Allowing yourself to let one slip-up derail you until the following Monday is a choice. Each meal you are presented with is a choice of what to eat. Slow down. Spend five minutes prior to eating to really think if that is the choice you want to make. If it is, don't feel guilty about it or shame yourself! If you decide it isn't worth it, stick to your plan instead! Things don't have to be a certain way every day for you to make progress. You just have to exercise discipline and moderation. That's it.

Setbacks will teach you a lesson every single time. Expect setbacks, because they are part of life. As far as my advice to overcome them, just keep moving forward. Even if it's light cardio, or even walking, just do something every day. Stay focused on your goals. I will not tell you to stay positive all the time, because that is impossible. Let yourself be pissed about the situation. Allow those feelings to exist and move through you. Being positive isn't always the answer, but being consistent is always forward motion!

10

THE BOXES WE PUT OURSELVES IN

The main reason people fail at losing weight or toning up is that they put themselves into a box, and their box has rules. Some of the most common weight loss misconceptions are:

- I have to eat five-six small meals a day to lose weight
- I can't eat carbs after 6pm
- I have to train seven days a week or I won't lose weight
- I have to starve myself to lose ten pounds
- I can't eat that many calories or I'll get fat
- I can't eat that much food, I'm not hungry often enough
- I don't have time to prep/eat six meals per day

Guess what? You don't have to do any of that. How many meals per day are feasible for you? Two? Lovely, do that. Breaking out of this mindset is harder than doing the actual work for a lot of people. Instead of just starting, many people sabotage themselves into thinking things have to be a certain way or nothing will work. For years I would start each Monday attempting perfection with my diet. I would be strict and rigid, only allowing certain items to land on my plate. By Wednesday, I inevitably made a mistake and then would consider the rest of the week a failure. "I'll start again next Monday," I'd tell myself.

This cycle continued for years. I was miserable and exhausted, I wasn't making progress, and at the end of each week, I would inevitably wonder, what was the fucking point?

It wasn't until I began changing the way I looked at these boxes I was shoving myself into that things changed. I started accepting my mistakes and getting right back on track with my meal plan. Another crucial step that cannot be overlooked is that I stopped allowing the voice in my head to verbally abuse me for my mistakes. I had to change my thought process. Food is food, not a mistake. Instead of mentally calculating how many miles I would have to run to burn off an ice cream sundae, shaming myself the whole way, I tried thinking, "Damn that was satisfying. I truly enjoyed that, and feel zero guilt. Back to my plan now!" I know this sounds simple, and it really is. You are almost always the one holding yourself back, my darlings. Not the fad diets. Not the ridiculous rules. Not the restrictions. You. You have convinced yourself that if you don't follow these rules that are beaten into your brain by society and mainstream media, that you will fail, but it's just not true.

Another massive falsehood about fitness is the amount of exercise you need to make progress. I used to think that if I wasn't going to be able to get in a two-hour, hardcore workout, I may as well not workout at all. I'd like to be the first to tell you that you don't have to exercise at all to make progress! I have dozens of clients who have never entered a gym, and have completely transformed their physique simply by following their meal plan (which by the way includes ice cream, tacos, and cocktails). Being freed from these mindsets transformed more than just my body, it transformed my mind. The more truth I found in the simplicity of the plan, and the more joy I found in helping others, the more I felt like the truest version of myself.

Six years later and I can finally say that I have stopped giving a fuck what everyone else thinks. Removing the dieting and fitness boxes led to removing the boxes in other areas of my life. I remember the barrage of judgments and questions that came when I first started getting my tattoos. "Are you really going to want that on your body when you are 80?" "Won't you regret getting that done?" "Tattoos take away your femininity, you know." "People won't want to work with you if you get more tattoos." Well guess what? I love my tattoos, and for anyone wondering, I am happy to tell you that I plan on getting more. Next up is the neck. Another thing that I quit caring about is what people thought about my Freddie Mercury obsession. I can't tell you how many times I've heard the words, "Maybe just don't share how much you like him, it makes you look obsessive." Hello? Did we just meet? Obsessive is my middle name.

One thing I have come to realize and accept is that when you are different, you make people feel uncomfortable. You are not conforming to what they believe is "normal." I've always known that I was not "normal," based on society's standards, and no matter how hard I tried, I was never able to fit into that mold. And trust me, I tried. I tried until I was so exhausted from trying to be someone else that I had no idea how to be myself. I hid the things I had done to achieve the body I have. I hid the things I was passionate about. I hid my addictions. I hid my self-loathing. I hid my alcohol consumption. I hid how I really felt about others. My feelings got tucked away at an early age and did not resurface until recently. I was so terrified to be myself out loud, that I lived miserably in my own fake existence. It almost cost me everything, and the only thing I was sure of was that I wasn't happy pretending anymore. I wanted to be liked for being Caroline, crazy and all.

11

TITS OUT

When you are aligned with your true self, your life begins. Time spent being anything other than your true self is distraction. This year I have had so many revelations about who I truly am, and while all of these positive changes were taking place in my mind, my physical health was dwindling more and more every day. I'd seen multiple doctors and specialists with no answers. As a last resort, I went to see an acupuncturist. As I filled out the intake forms I caught myself checking off so many symptoms that it was alarming. The nurse who listened to me and assessed my symptoms, said, "You know, for someone who appears to be very healthy and in shape, you are extremely unhealthy." It was like a punch in my gut. Hearing those words left me with more fear and confusion.

Even though I was dealing with unexplained, debilitating symptoms, I still hadn't made the connection that my breast implants could be the cause of them. They were approaching the thirteen year mark, and I knew it was time to do something, so I booked a consultation to freshen them up. During my consultation there was a pit in my stomach the entire time. I felt unsure, but I said nothing. I chose silicon implants because I had saline and hated the ripple feeling they had. If I was going to do this again, I wanted to get the mac daddy of implants, so I booked the surgery for six weeks later. Each day after booking my surgery I woke up feeling unsure of my decision. I went to my pre-op appointment and expressed concerns to my nurse about switching out my saline implants for silicone. As I sat there reading over the waiver, the words "these implants could potentially cause cancer" flashed before my eyes. I literally choked. My gut instinct was screaming at me. I couldn't get those words out of my head. Having kids made me think more deeply about the decision I had made. Was this going to be worth it if I got cancer and died? Was having bigger boobs worth my family losing their wife and mother? These are the thoughts that were swirling around my mind, preventing me from being engaged in any discussion that was going on around me. I had to figure out what I wanted to do. Me. Nobody else. So I did what I always do when it comes to big decisions, I made a joke.

I laughingly asked Pooh Bear what he would think about me just removing my implants altogether. He was confused, almost dumbfounded, at this suggestion, as I had just attended my pre op, and dropped $11k that afternoon on new and improved tits. He tried to make sense of the question for at least an hour, and then we began having a real discussion about me cancelling my surgery. In the end, he expressed to me that whatever decision I made he would be in full support of. I had mosquito bites when he met me, so he certainly didn't marry me for these things. I felt comfortable making the decision to cancel my surgery once I had him on board, and I knew what my sister would (and did) have to say about it ("You never should have gotten them in the first place, idiot. Rip 'em out.").

My nurse was so understanding and assured me that if I was even 1% unsure that I should not go forward with the surgery. I decided to take some time to think about what I wanted to do, whether that meant scheduling an explant immediately or waiting. The next evening I saw a Facebook post from a good friend/former co-worker from Hooters, regarding her explant. I immediately sent her a message asking her why she chose to do it. What she shared with me was the catalyst for my own decision to explant. As she described her symptoms, I got chills all over my body. I had damn near all of the symptoms she was describing. The puzzle was coming together. My intuition had been screaming at me at that consult, and until this moment I didn't know why. She explained to me that if I chose to move forward with the explant, that it was critical to choose a microsurgeon who specializes in the en bloc procedure. The en bloc procedure involves leaving the capsule tissue intact on the breast implant and cutting around it without disrupting the capsule or implant. The capsules are the things your body naturally forms around the implants in order to protect your body. The irony of the capsules "protecting" me is not lost on me. Removing the capsules with the implants is done to avoid contamination that may lead to breast implant illness (BII). En bloc is a delicate and meticulous procedure. She shared her surgeon's name and number with me and I called the next day to schedule a consultation for an explant. My explant consultation felt so different. I felt sure that this was what I was supposed to be doing. The sense of peace and comfort I felt after making the decision was amazing.

After making the decision to explant and speaking with my doctor, I started to wonder how many of the health issues I'd experienced over the last couple years might be related to my implants. I sat down to map out some of the unexplained symptoms I'd been experiencing and see if they lined up.

✓ Excessive swallowing/trouble swallowing

✓ Headaches

✓ Joint pain

✓ Random bouts of nausea

✓ Ear pain

✓ Throat clearing

✓ Anxiety

✓ The feeling that I'm choking

✓ Bouts of depression/suicidal thoughts

✓ Exhaustion/fatigue

✓ Abdominal pain

✓ Heart palpitations

✓ Skin rashes

✓ Low libido

✓ Shooting pain in breasts

✓ Overactive bladder

✓ Mood swings

✓ Forgetfulness/foggy head

These symptoms started about two years ago and have progressively gotten worse over the past six months. The exhaustion was so real that I could barely get a workout in, and the choking sensation was also a really fun time. It has happened in the middle of the night a few times now, and it is absolutely terrifying. You think "this is it, this is the moment I am going to die." I started to wonder if some of what I thought were side effects of the steroids were actually BII, and I began to have hope that my voice would return once I get these toxic bags taken out of my chest. The things we do to look a certain way and receive approval from others is just outrageous. I felt like I was heading home to the real Caroline by making the decision to get them out. I never thought I would utter these words, but I was so ready to be flat chested again.

I was always flat-chested growing up. I was called all the names in the book by the boys, including my personal favorite "mosquito bites." It tortured me that I wasn't developing as fast as the other girls. I was the last one to get my period, the last to get boobs, and I looked like a boy. When I made the cheer squad there was a very clear shift in me feeling more girly. I suddenly started getting attention from the boys and it felt amazing, I won't lie. Living for the approval of others started here and lasted until this very year as I grappled with the decision to remove my implants. I was terrified of what my husband would think. Listen, I know Pooh Bear loves me unconditionally and supported my decision, but I was so scared that he would look at me differently if I had nothing there again. That was a large part of why I hesitated for so long on the decision. What was strange is that I felt a deep sense of knowing that they needed to come out. But the fear of what others would think and the thought of what I would look like without them were the only things holding me back. It really is silly when you think about it.

Even as I have been growing my company, I have had to overcome not feeling authentic. I was working with a marketing company to expand CWC. We were launching a huge campaign which revolved around donuts. I felt so inauthentic. Do I love donuts? Yes, I do. But the things they were asking me to do felt so forced. I felt like I was being shoved into a box, and you all know my thoughts on that. It was a recipe for failure. I was doing everything they asked, pushing, hustling, but the momentum just ceased. Nobody was even asking me about CWC anymore, much less signing up. And guess what? I was exhausted. The harder I worked, the harder it got. I thought the more work you put in, the easier it would be, but that just wasn't the case when I was being managed. I was burning the candle at both ends and finally had to put the flames out. I chose to part ways with them amicably, but they still support me and my company to this very day.

I ended up reaching out to an old friend from middle school, Sarah. We never hung out when we attended school together, but she was a client of mine and she was launching her own mentoring business and so I asked her about it one day. She told me that we could begin working together, but her one stipulation was that I had to go back to being myself. I laughed and replied "What do you mean?" She said "The donut stuff has to go, it isn't you." I had two feelings at the same time: relief and an epiphany. That's why my business had become crickets overnight! I wasn't sharing what they were used to seeing and what drew them to me initially: me!

In the same moment I felt immediate relief that I no longer had to do cold calls (I'd literally rather eat broccoli than make cold calls), make scripted videos, have someone monitoring my Instagram account, randomly messaging women from my inbox, only to receive hate mail in reply every day. These tactics may work wonders for some business models, but they definitely did not for CWC. I built my business on sharing my story and being 100% true to my followers, and now I could go back to doing just that. I immediately began being myself again, and the interest grew almost immediately. Since that shift, the Community has exploded. We are now over 2,000 members, I have three coaches under me, I am writing my second book, and I have a podcast as well. It is crazy to think that Sarah and I have not even been working together for a year yet and all of these insane changes have taken place. And not only have I implemented them into my business, but my personal life as well. I have gotten so good at listening to my intuition and following it that it was truly what led me to making the decision to remove my breast implants. Doing this has allowed me to reach so many women, and connect with them on another level. I documented my entire journey on my social media platforms as well as my CWC Podcast, holding nothing back and showing my girls each step of my journey.

The number of women still reaching out to me to talk about BII is alarming. Most women are desperate to get theirs removed, but financially unable to. Others are terrified of having surgery now that they are older, and some are simply scared to be flat-chested again. This is exactly why I decided to share my story. The realities of BII, both big and small, are not discussed enough. I lost countless nights of sleep due to the throat clearing issue. My primary doctor thought I was crazy when I told her about it. She looked at me as if she had never heard anyone say these things. She suggested that I see my dentist (add one more person to the list who thinks I'm a lunatic).

As I got closer and closer to my surgery, I felt like I was running on fumes. I was struggling to get my errands run, keep my business going, and take care of my family. That's when I knew something had to change. Even now, looking back at how poorly I was functioning is overwhelming. Thoughts on why I chose to get them in the first place bombarded my mind. As I reflect on that time, I guess the desire to have bigger breasts stemmed from being made fun of so much as a child. I was a size AA, so when I say I was flat chested, I am not exaggerating. At that time in my life, in my mid-twenties, they made me feel sexier and more confident. Now that I'm older and have children, my priorities have changed. I need my fucking health back. I need to be there for my family. I want to workout and leave feeling better than when I walked in, instead of feeling like my workouts are sucking the life out of me. When I say "I'm taking my life back," it's the truth.

*****

The week leading up to my surgery I experienced the worst anxiety of my entire life. I was literally counting down the minutes. I was terrified that something would happen that would cancel my surgery. I was terrified to go anywhere or touch things, for fear that I may catch something and get sick and not be able to have the surgery. My anxiety was so bad that I started experiencing physical reactions that weren't real. I felt my throat itching, and thought "this is it, I'm getting sick and won't be able to get these things out." I avoided the gym that whole week. I cleaned everything at my house just to keep my mind off of it. That week felt like an entire year. But once the day came, I was completely at ease. I knew they had to come out. I was certain that they were the cause of so many of my health issues, and I was fucking right.

I woke up from surgery feeling like a million dollars. Obviously I was high as hell, but I could breathe. I could actually take a full breath without having to brace myself and concentrate. The difference in how I felt coming out of this surgery compared to having them put in was night and day. Even with anesthesia, I was alert and remembered the conversation I had with the post op nurse. I remember seeing Pooh Bear walk into the recovery room. I'm just now approaching three weeks post op and to say I feel like a completely different human is an understatement. Here are the things that have changed so far:

✓ My bizarre ear pain is completely gone. It constantly felt muffled and full, and it doesn't anymore.

✓ My hair feels different, fuller

✓ My skin tone and face shape has changed dramatically

✓ My nails are growing rapidly

✓ My appetite has returned; I have a desire for food again

✓ My energy is back. Even in recovery I have more energy than I've had in years

✓ Suicidal/terribly anxious thoughts racing through my brain are gone

✓ I feel like Caroline again

✓ The brain fog is getting better every day

✓ The throat clearing is getting much better

✓ I no longer feel like I'm choking at random times

✓ Swallowing is getting easier

✓ Headaches are gone

✓ I don't pee 38 times a day

Now you all know by now that I am well versed in vagina struggles. An overactive bladder is one of the main symptoms of BII. Almost every woman I have spoken to has experienced it. It's like having a urinary tract infection without the burning sensation (super fun). You literally pee every ten minutes regardless of how much liquid you consume. This issue was probably the most disruptive overall to my day-to-day life. I would have to interrupt meetings multiple times just to run to the bathroom and empty what little urine was in my bladder. The most irritating part was the sensation that you never fully emptied your bladder. I saw my urologist more times in the past year and a half than I'd like to admit. He suggested doing scopes, different medications, and even did ultrasounds on my kidneys multiple times. One week prior to my explant, he officially diagnosed me with an overactive bladder. I looked him in the eyes and begged him to tell me if he thought that this could potentially be related to my breast implants. He gave me the stock response that every other doctor always gave me which was basically, there's no way of knowing. I am ridiculously elated to report to you guys that just thirteen days after having my explant, my bladder issues have resolved about 92%. I can actually drink lots of fluids now and not have to run to the bathroom every ten minutes, and it is the greatest feeling in the entire world. Not to mention I can add more things on my to-do list now that don't involve being near a porta-john.

Prior to my surgery I can remember running and running and running and feeling so tired, but never feeling like I was doing enough. Now everything has slowed down to a snail's pace because I need help with everything. I need help opening my car door, pulling something from the top shelf in the fridge, etc. What's interesting is that I'm realizing that I'm just as productive, running at about 1/100 of the pace. I know it sounds crazy, but I feel like my life has started all over again.

12

LOSS

After my surgery, we moved into a mobile home and got to work building our dream house. The first week was stressful, but I stayed on track. I got a gazillion steps in, and felt so good. Since my explant, my energy has been through the roof. To live the past two fucking years feeling like I was dying a slow, miserable death with no answers, to now feeling like I have my life and will to live back has been so amazing. One day I actually hit 17,000 steps. I felt so good. Even though we were moving, living in a tight ass space with our crazy kids and three dogs, we got it done and I wasn't exhausted. Life was good, and I finally felt as if things were going back to normal. Then Halloween arrived.

We were wrapping up dinner when I heard my husband ask, "What's wrong with Lou?" I looked over and my perfect girl, our little french bulldog was lying on the ground, in a very weird position. She looked like she was paralyzed and her eyes looked empty. She was still breathing, but we assumed maybe some of her food got stuck in her throat so my husband turned her on her side and checked her mouth. Nothing. She then began to gasp for air and lost control of her bladder and bowels. I was screaming at this point, and so were the kids. Josh was trying to focus on figuring out how to help her and picked her up to take her outside so that he could do that. I immediately knew this wasn't good. I felt helpless and panicked. I heard my son scream and I looked over to see him staring out the front window. It was at this point I knew that she was gone. She was my perfect girl and now in a matter of seconds she had been ripped away from me. It seemed so unfair. I became angry.

My mom loves to tell stories about what an angry child I was. I remember the rage that was deep inside of me from a very young age. I still don't know why it's there, or where it stems from but as an adult I have gotten pretty good at controlling it. Meditation helps, deep breathing helps, and steering my focus off of the thing that's making me angry seems to help as well. But I couldn't escape this. It was all around me. The pain, the anger, the terror, the sadness, it left me lifeless. My brain has been trying to make sense of it all and it just can't. Our vet said that she could have thrown a blood clot, or that it could have been a heart attack. Either way, it doesn't solve anything.

The pain was unlike anything I'd experienced in so long that I lost control. I stress ate, I drank, and I didn't give a fuck. I coped by numbing, and I had gotten really good at not doing that. I feel like a failure, a fraud. I had nothing in me to give. How would I even begin to offer up any help to my clients? The expectations that we place on ourselves are what crush us, but we often forget that we are in full control of the entire machine.

In the beginning of my transformation it was so easy to motivate others. I was putting in the work, nothing was getting in my way, and if something did, I just pushed forward anyway. I am currently trying to tap back into this. I have been trying to hop back in the saddle for so long now, but I feel like I keep getting bucked off. After Lou died, I just wanted to lie on the ground and give up. But I couldn't. I had to hold out hope that, if I just kept moving, things would begin to turn back around. I needed them to turn around. Before, when I was stressed, I was in shape and felt good about myself, so it didn't affect me like it was now. I had lost progress, and was not comfortable in my skin again. It was a terrible feeling. I tell my clients to love their bodies every step of the way, but I sometimes don't, and post-injury and post-op, this was one of those times.

Not being able to really train over the past two years definitely contributed to these feelings. Realizing that I needed my implants out in order for my body to be working in my favor again, having the surgery, and recovering from the surgery also contributed. As a result, my body fat increased and my muscle mass decreased. This directly affected my mood, and I knew it. I knew what I needed to do moving forward, and I wasn't going to stop. I know that setbacks will continue to happen, but I also know that there is only one thing that will truly destroy me, and that's quitting.

I have spent the last few months trying to figure out myself all over again. Why do I find so much comfort in rage and anger? It always feels so safe. Being strong and doing the right thing has never come easy to me, I always just succumb to the anger and allow it to wrap me up like a cocoon. This past year I had a breakthrough in one of my therapy sessions when I was trying to figure out the answer to this. It suddenly hit me when my therapist asked me what feeling I got when I would dive straight to the worst case scenarios in any given situation. After thinking about it, I told her that it made me feel safe. But why on earth would that make anyone feel safe? When I look back at my childhood, I realize that this is what my mother did (and still does). Sometimes I can't even speak to her if I am concerned about something because I know her brain will automatically jump to the worst possible scenario and then I begin spiralling as well, worrying about her manifesting terrible outcomes on my behalf. The anger, fear, and doomsday mindset are comforting because they feel like home. If I know up front the worst that can happen, then nothing will shock me or scare me because I will have already imagined the worst happening. So when I lost my Lou, that was one of my worst possible scenarios playing out right in front of my eyes, and I couldn't stop it.

So in perfect form, I am finishing this book full circle, having turned to food to cope again, and inviting alcohol back to the game as well, letting it whisper to me, begging to take the pain away. That voice came back so fast that I didn't even have time to prepare myself for it. For anyone else, to cope with alcohol may be just fine. But for me, I know that it is a slippery slope, and one that would be very hard to stop, and I didn't want to get on that ride again. I texted my sister and told her that I was considering taking up alcoholism again. I mean, it was so much fun the first time around, why not give it another go? The concern was there, but she told me to cope however I wanted to, but to know that she would be checking in on me over the next few weeks to make sure I wasn't lost in a sea of booze. She knows from extensive experience that ultimatums and shame only make the problem worse, and having the "pass" to hit the bottle somehow helped. I came home from work that night and went straight for the tequila.

I didn't even bother making a drink. I just shot it straight from the bottle. I could sense the concern brewing in my husband when he walked in and said, "That is not the answer." I replied "Well nothing else is either so what does it even matter?" Except I know what matters now. My life matters. I have a beautiful family, a gorgeous piece of land where we are about to build another dream home, a farm with a bunch of goofy, deliciously cute animals, and a super supportive husband. I couldn't see all of this when I was dealing with my postpartum depression back in 2013, but I can see it so clearly now, and I know I have the choice to go down the hill, or to hike back up. I could choose to drown myself in alcohol and food, numbing the fuck out of myself, or I could let myself grieve, and then choose to fall back on the coping mechanism that got me off the booze the first time: exercise. So after a couple of weeks of a food and alcohol free-for-all, I went back to the gym, I blasted Freddie Mercury, and I worked my fucking ass off. It felt so good, so cathartic. I thought of Lou the entire time and it was exactly what I needed. Knowing that I had the choice is what made all the difference, and that is what I wanna drive home now that we are nearing the end of this book: if you don't like your life, you have the permission to change it. You have full control over every choice that you make every single day. You have full control over every reaction you have to any given situation.

A close friend of mine once told me, mid-breakdown, to "triage your life." It stuck with me and now it is on a post-it on my desk. It's perfect if you think about it. These days we are on full alert with everything in real time. We see everyone we know on social media every single day, living their lives right alongside them, constantly comparing even if we don't mean to. It's complete sensory overload for me sometimes and there are days I want to delete all of my social media accounts and just disappear, but I can't. I have a company that requires me to be on social media every single day. I will never complain about that because my job breathes life into me and I never want to be doing anything else.

So I can triage my life. I can take breaks, no matter how long. I don't want to be all or nothing like I was before. I want to utilize that discipline muscle that I've worked so hard to strengthen. Muscle memory is real and progress happens fast, so as long as I can get back on track for just a few weeks, I know I'll be back. You don't have to give it 100%, seven days a week to see change. The secret is doing what you can every single day and not letting anything keep you lying on the floor, no matter how physically or mentally challenging it is to get up and get going again.

I have spent the past eight years strengthening my discipline muscle, and as a result my self confidence has soared. When you build up your self confidence, you act differently. You become the best version of yourself. At thirty-eight years old I've finally become the woman I always wanted to be. I am strong, not only physically but mentally. I have created a life that I love. I love waking up every day and getting to go to "work." I don't dread the days anymore. Committing to working on my body six years ago, and to put down the bottle when things got tough, led me to the realization that there is a better way to live than being on a diet, and ultimately led me to create this Community that teaches real women with real food cravings how to enjoy their lives and love their bodies.

13

JOURNALING, MEDITATION, AND THERAPY

You choose your story. I think the hardest part of getting through a shitty situation, or getting started with no motivation, is knowing that deep down you are in full control of both. I've always said that it is scary and empowering all at the same time that it's completely up to you. You can choose to let that terrify and cripple you, or you can choose to let it ignite something inside of you to put forth the effort to change. Believe me when I tell you that I have been knocked down more times than I can count over the past two years, but I have yet to give up. I may have given up on some days, some weeks, hell even some months, but I haven't completely thrown in the towel altogether like I used to.

Sharing my shit has been the one thing that has helped me to connect with my clients over the years. In the beginning, when I was still navigating this course, albeit poorly and all by myself, I was exhausted every day. I would go to the gym and try to post on my Instagram story about my amazing workout, but some days I didn't even have the energy to warm up. I felt like I was just making it through each day. It was a combination of things, such as feeling burnt out with my marketing strategies, CWC growing (which was amazing, but also overwhelming), and ultimately I was running on fumes and not taking care of myself like I would daily preach to my clients. What a fuckin' hypocrite! So I reached out to a couple of coaches I followed on Instagram. I had been following them for years and they seemed to coach very similarly to me. No crash diets, just realistic approaches from people who seemed to truly care about their clients. I signed up and told them that my goals were not necessarily physical, but more mental. I wanted to have a grasp on my thoughts and feelings,

I also needed my energy to increase if I wanted to continue growing my business. The first thing they suggested was journaling and meditation. What?! Why? I immediately told them that I did not have time for those things (what a fucking twat I was). They laughed and told me that my response made me sound like someone who absolutely needed journaling and meditation. Fine. I agreed to try it, but I wasn't going to like it.

The journaling was hard. I was supposed to write down things I loved about myself, things I wanted out of life, and specifically things I was not (to help retrain my brain out of behaviors I wasn't fond of in myself--such as being reactive). I remember trying to write "I am not reactive." Man, my hand could not even move the pen across the paper. I didn't believe it, so how would I be able to write it? My coach told me to keep writing it over and over until it became something my brain believed. And that is what I did. It's been six months and I am extremely less reactive now. The brain is a funny thing. I never even thought twice about the things I was feeding my brain on a daily basis, but that's also why I was so unhappy for so long. I truly believed, and constantly reminded myself daily, that I wasn't good enough. And the sad thing was that it was all bullshit. I have learned that not only am I good enough, but I can do anything that I set my mind to. What are you saying to yourself every day? Deep inside where you know that nobody can hear you. Here are some things I used to say to myself:

1. "I am fat."

2. "I am not good enough."

3. "I don't contribute to my family."

4. "I need ___ and ___ for this person to like me."

5. "I need to make more money."

6. “I can’t diet, I love food too much.”

7. “I’m not as pretty as _____”

8. “I am angry.”

9. “I hate my stomach.”

These were just a few of the mortifying things I said to myself on a daily basis. On the outside, none of my friends or family would have ever known. I was programming my brain to keep me in a state of failure, never feeling good enough for being me. If I wanted to be great, I had to be someone else. But that was such a giant load of shit, and if you were to read my list, I bet you would tell me the same thing. Just as if I were to read your list, I would immediately begin to tell you that those things are not true. I would start commenting on all the good things about you, and how you are literally holding yourself back from being great with these lies you keep telling yourself.

I am going to dedicate this section for you to practice a journal session of your very own, and you are not allowed to say you can’t think of anything!

Write down ten things you are grateful for:

1.____

2.____

3.____

4.____

5.____

6.____

7.____________________________________

8.____________________________________

9.____________________________________

10.____________________________________

Now write ten things you love about yourself:

1.____________________________________

2.____________________________________

3.____________________________________

4.____________________________________

5.____________________________________

6.____________________________________

7.____________________________________

8.____________________________________

9.____________________________________

10.____________________________________

Meditation was something that honestly made me laugh when I thought about executing it. Should I sit on my patio in the morning with the birds chirping, hands on my knees, with my index finger touching my thumb, humming while my children perform a full on WWE fight in the background? Surely no one really expected me to do this. I had to figure out how to make this work for me and my schedule. Much like following a meal plan, exercising, or anything in life, you have to make it work for you. One of the biggest obstacles that hold people back is believing that things have to be done a certain way. They don't.

My meditation sessions look like this: drop the kids off at school, park my car in a parking lot, turn on Theta waves on YouTube, lean back in my seat, and zone out. When I meditate I cannot turn off my thoughts. They actually begin to race more. So I have to just focus on each breath I take. I breathe in for three seconds and out for four-five. Focusing on this forces my brain to release all those thoughts about nachos and tacos that are floating around automatically so I can fully engage. I like to meditate immediately after journaling because all of my goals and aspirations are fresh in my mind, and I find it easier to envision all of them. The first time I meditated, I had a huge breakthrough. I literally saw all of the things I wanted for my life flashing before the inside of my eyelids. It was amazing. Things I wanted for my family, my career, my life. They were all there. I cannot explain the feeling but it made my skin feel like it was tingling. So whatever it looks like for you, make it work. Don't try to fit it into an unrealistic box or it's gonna feel like a chore and you won't do it. Check out the YouTube link on the back of the book for some great meditation resources!

*****

I want to preface this section by admitting that therapy is a subject that I never would have imagined being in any book I wrote. Ever. Therapy was for weak people. Therapy was for crybabies. And I was neither of those things. Except I was.

The journaling and meditation were helping, but the missing piece of the puzzle was therapy. I was on the phone with my sister one day, having one of my usual breakdowns and she had had enough. She screamed at me to go see a therapist and I fucking lost it. I screamed back at her, accused her of thinking I was weak, and hung up, swearing I would never talk to her again. I was over her. Done.

Do you see how much I needed therapy in my life? I knew deep down I needed it, but I was terrified. Emily had sent me the information of three local therapists a year prior (that she had extensively researched based off of 1. If they specialized in what she thought was wrong with me, 2. If they were taking new patients, and 3. Whether or not she thought I'd like their face). I pulled up the first lady from that list, googled her number, and called her office right there on the spot, before I could change my mind (don't tell my sister that). Her assistant booked me for the following day, and the rest is history. I was still experiencing erratic thoughts from time to time, and as I sat down on her couch that first day I told her that I wanted to "feel less crazy." I just wanted to feel normal. What would it be like to finally feel normal?

We have been working together since March and I wish I would have started 20 years ago. I have had breakthroughs about my OCD, my anxiety, my need for approval, and we haven't even scratched the surface yet. One thing I have had to accept is that I will forever be "working" on myself, which sucks if I'm being completely honest. Sometimes it's too much. Sometimes just getting up and doing the day-to-day shit is too much for me to handle. But that is fucking life, and that is something I pass onto my clients daily. They get started, get a good solid week under their belt, and then life happens. They say "maybe now isn't the right time." Wrong. There is never a good time to do anything. Life will always come along and blindside your ass with something, so you better just learn to deal with it and keep moving. Movement is medicine.

Journaling, meditation, and therapy have made me feel far less crazy than I ever imagined I could feel, and that is something I can't put a price on. Complete the following questions to determine what might be holding you back from reaching your goals!

What are the things holding you back from living your best life?

1.____

2.____

3.____

4.____

5.____

What are some of the things you struggle with in regards to reaching your physical goals?

1.____

2.____

3.____

4.____

5.____

Now write down what you think might be the answers to each thing you listed in the above question. And yes, you do have the answers within yourself!

1.____

2.____

3.____

4.____

5.____

"Success is the sum of small efforts, repeated day in and day out."

Robert Collier

Lastly, I want you to write down ten things you want out of your life, or how you want your life to look. It can be crazy as hell, the wilder the better, but if it's in your head, write it down!

1.____

2.____

3.____

4.____

5.____

6.____

7.____

8.____

9.____

10.____

I hope you enjoyed *Back for Seconds*! I loved writing it and sharing all of these stories with you. Scan the QR code below to check out my Linktree, where you can join our free Facebook group, Community with Caroline, visit my website, subscribe to the CWC Podcast, get your copy of my first book, *One More Bite*, contact me directly, follow me on Instagram, and check out some of my must-haves on Amazon. If you complete the tasks in this book, we would love for you to post about your experience in our Community!

IN MEMORY OF MY PERFECT GIRL, LOU.

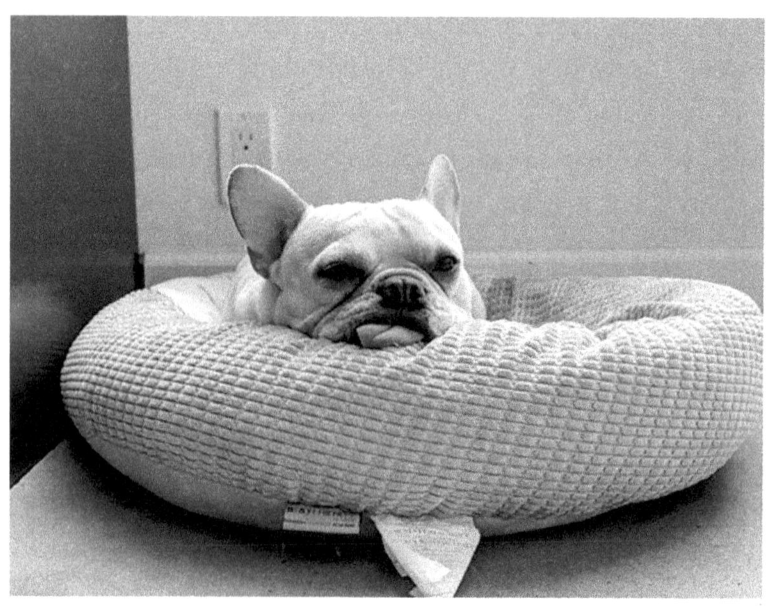

CPSIA information can be obtained
at www.ICGtesting.com
Printed in the USA
LVHW010021220921
698400LV00003B/14

9 780578 985374